# Lost for Words

# Lost for Words

## Talking about Loss in Childbearing

### What to Say When You Don't Know What to Say

Sue Mack and Julie Tucker

*ISBN 9781708371142*

*For all those who have experienced loss in pregnancy*

.

# Table of Contents

# Introduction

Everyone with experience in the helping professions has had to manage the pain, and often the lasting effects, of loss. This is particularly true for those working with pregnant and postpartum women and their partners. Figures from the UK government national statistics for 2016 show there are just under 200,000 terminations each year in the UK, and a fairly steady number of 17 babies are stillborn or die shortly after birth *each day*. Around 20% of pregnancies end in miscarriage. There are also unknown numbers of very early miscarriages which may be unacknowledged or unrecorded, some of which may be seen in GP practices. There are around 50,000 inpatient admissions to hospitals in the UK every year for early pregnancy loss.

This book explores the needs of the clients, those close to them and the staff working with them through their childbearing experience. It offers information on how to approach the difficult conversations the professionals often need to have. It is intended as a handbook to consult on particular areas of loss and as a guide to dealing with loss in general. Some information is repeated in relation to different parts of the journey of pregnancy and childbirth. It may be useful for training, for Continuing Professional Development groups (CPDs) and as a signpost towards Personal Development Plans (PDPs). We will explore the professional guidelines supporting midwives, nurses and doctors, as well as ethical considerations around pregnancy and loss.

As we undertook our research for the book, it soon became apparent that much of the information we wanted to provide was from research completed some time ago. We have used that which we feel is relevant, even if it is not current. We hope readers will be inspired to undertake their own research, developing and updating the information on this very important, but under-researched, topic.

The losses we are dealing with may be a woman's (and her family's) actual loss of a pregnancy, of a child or the mother herself; or the loss of the anticipated experience of the perfect baby. Pregnancy changes everything. It changes how a woman feels about herself and her future, how other people regard her, and her place in society. Whether a pregnancy is planned, unplanned, wanted or unwanted, the woman will be changed by it. Loss in pregnancy or childbirth brings further change.

Each stage of pregnancy brings different expectations and needs for information, interaction and care. The experiences that each individual client and professional bring to their preparation for a pregnancy and afterwards can have both positive and negative effects. The more we understand about our own needs, expectations and prejudices, the more we are able to support one another and to communicate clearly. The stages we will consider are: the pressure to become pregnant and decisions about keeping the pregnancy; early pregnancy, screening and the second trimester; the third trimester, preparing for birth and after delivery; and considering the psychological and support needs around loss (actual or felt) at each of these stages.

We have chapters on the three trimesters and the different issues faced at those times, as well as the general areas of loss, communication and counselling. We want this book to be a useful aid in managing the challenges of loss and anticipated loss; and the experiences that these women, their partners and families may have. Our aim is to help those seeking the right words in various situations that regularly confront nurses, midwives and all those working with childbearing women. We want to help those professionals wanting to inform and support clients experiencing loss, and to support the staff themselves to better understand loss and its effects.

Support organisations can offer tremendous help at all stages of a loss. Being in touch with others who have had the same or a similar experience can help people to feel 'normal', to reassure them about their feelings and sometimes about the future. We will explore the use of support groups and social media in this context and the value of both personal and remote support.

We shall see from the research that both staff and clients feel better able to cope with loss at all stages of pregnancy if they are informed and feel confident in discussing the loss and the feelings it arouses in everyone. This can be a traumatic event for anyone involved and a challenging area of practice. We look at how to avoid words and phrases that could potentially trigger distress for clients and staff, and to say the words that are helpful and supportive. The case studies from our own practice are intended as illustrations to help provide ideas on how to tackle particular areas and to suggest ways of approaching these conversations.

We hope this book will help with those times when we, as professionals, really do not know what to say and feel afraid of saying the wrong thing. It is not intended to make huge changes in practice, especially given the limited time we know staff have available to spend with clients; but to consider a way of thinking and of interacting with them that relates to their thoughts and feelings at a crucial time of loss or potential loss. We often refer to midwives and nurses, but we do intend the book to be useful for all staff working with women and their babies.

We explore models of loss and grieving in relation to pregnancy and childbirth and how these relate to actual practice and care. We will consider the research and use the knowledge we have gained over many years of practice and teaching. The experiences of midwives, doctors and other professionals, as well as their clients, all contribute to understanding the needs of patients, families and staff and the difficulties they face when discussing these painful and distressing experiences and decisions.

We deal with the difficult area of breaking bad news with empathy and genuineness, without it becoming too distressing for the professional and their colleagues; and so that they feel they are offering support and help to all those involved. We do not expect the professionals to become counsellors but using some of the principles of counselling may help in these difficult areas of practice. Based on research, good practice and our own experience, we will examine the principles of good communication, particularly in a new, frightening or unexpected situation.

Clients and staff may look to the experience, knowledge and support of others and increasingly, digital media, to help them to understand what is happening and how to manage it. If communication is supportive, understandable and consonant with our beliefs, everyone can feel safer and better cared for.

Loss is universal but there are differences in how different cultures and religions approach the subject. We also address this and offer coping strategies and support in cross-cultural and differing religious situations. We are concerned with care for the caregivers and we know from our own practice that there are limited options for learning in the workplace. Finding the support and space to discuss this sensitive area can be difficult, so staff may hold onto their anxieties and vulnerabilities. The culture is not always amenable to sharing and learning from others. Even the good can get lost. In acknowledging the experiences of others, we hope to open up conversations on this stressful topic.

Research and our experience suggest a common need expressed by clients, families, staff and society for clear, honest and genuine communication when there are difficult decisions and outcomes to manage[1]. These needs are defined by our expectations, experiences and the norms of our society. This is true not just for the clients, but also for the caregivers. We are all influenced by what has happened to us in the past and by our expectations of pregnancy and childbirth. The fear of loss can be a very powerful one for those who have previously experienced it. This may be directly related to a pregnancy or a child, but may also be part of another, unresolved or hidden, loss from the past; and it may not be obvious as a cause of anxiety or depression to the client, her partner or those close to her.

Partners, families and social groups are inseparable. They interact constantly and affect one another. We will explore how this in turn affects good communication, using real examples from our own practice, with some details changed to ensure confidentiality. In considering effective communications between the families and the professionals, we also acknowledge the importance of not only the words used but also the difficulties that can arise when English is either not spoken within the family or is the second language.

Throughout this book you will hear the two voices of the authors contributing their knowledge and extensive practical experience of midwifery and counselling to support all those affected by loss. We acknowledge that beginning these conversations causes stress and carries with it anxiety. We want to provide help with those difficult and challenging experiences in practice when we are not sure how best to offer helpful support and guidance, because we have all, at times, found ourselves 'lost for words'.

# Acknowledgements

Sue and Julie would like to acknowledge the following people for the support they provided during the writing of this book:

John Mack for his wise words and unwavering support. Judith Harvey for reading the manuscript and offering valid and helpful comments to help us complete the book. Izzy Aungier and her friends for their valuable input. Louise Jennet for always being there with professional advice during the writing process. Suzanne Wilton for invaluable help with editing and proofreading. Steve Holden for investing his time, commitment and superior technical skills in helping to get the book published. Jane Arezina for giving her permission for her work to be quoted.

This book came out of the work we have done together supporting staff, women and their families who have experienced loss professionally and personally. Thank you to them all for trusting in us to help them by talking about their experiences. They remain anonymous, as we have used fictitious names throughout the book.

# About the Authors

Sue Mack is a counsellor and psychotherapist who has worked for many years in the NHS with women and families in the area of termination and early pregnancy loss. In her private practice and in private hospitals she has specialised in working with women who have experienced loss and bereavement and with people suffering depressive illness.

Julie Tucker qualified as a midwife in 1975 and worked through all areas of maternity, both in hospital and private practice. She transferred her skills to caring for those with fertility problems and also qualified as a counsellor. She worked as a fertility counsellor in many units whilst continuing to be a midwife. In the latter part of her career, she became a Bereavement Midwife, which bought many of her learned skills together.

Together, Sue and Julie co-wrote *Fertility Counselling*, published in 1999.

# Foreword

Birth is a usually considered a joyful event. But sometimes things go wrong and the outcome is not as wished for. As a midwife I have had the joy and privilege of sharing in many happy arrivals, but often it is the sad outcomes that provide the challenge and opportunity to provide meaningful care that resonates for both healthcare practitioners and the families for years to come.

Much has been written about experience of pregnancy loss, more usually from the family's perspective. For the healthcare professional it is also a difficult experience, and we are not always certain how best we can offer support. This handbook sets out guidance for what to say when we simply don't know what to say.

Financial constraints mean there is a dearth of professional counselling services available for families and it is often the first line carers, such as sonographers, fertility nurses, doctors and midwives who are the only source of support, often with limited time. Breaking bad news is within their remit, and the training is limited.

Each individual will experience the grief—or even relief—of loss in a unique way. With over fifty years of work in fertility, midwifery and birth work between them, the authors have drawn on their vast knowledge and expertise to produce guidance for both the novice and experienced alike.

There are clearly-defined sections covering diagnoses of anomalies, early and late miscarriage, stillbirth and life beyond. Each chapter uses extensive case studies drawn from their own practice and gives wise guidance for healthcare staff working with pregnancy loss, spanning the earliest days of conception to full term stillbirth.

This is the ultimate and much needed handbook for student midwives, gynaecology nurses, sonographers and indeed any student, qualified staff or support carers working in the field of fertility, midwifery and obstetrics.

**Louise Jennett**
Lecturer in Midwifery, *University of Brighton*
Professional Midwifery Advocate,
*Brighton and Sussex University Hospitals NHS Trust*

# 1: Loss and Grieving

*The grieving process; the process of mourning; cultural differences in mourning; siblings and loss; relationships with professionals; the end of mourning; investing in another relationship.*

Loss is universal and inevitable, but no-one is ever quite prepared for it or quite the same afterwards. It brings about change sometimes in how we live our lives, in our relationships and our thoughts about the future; and always in our expectations. No one person's loss is the same as another's and there is no one way to grieve. Those who have lost someone may feel a sense of unreality, of anger, sadness, helplessness and any combination of these things and more. It may be difficult to observe and to be close to but the support or lack of support that someone receives near the time of the loss can affect how they manage their feelings in the future. For example, it may be frightening or feel shameful that you are angry with the child who has died, or with your partner; but clients can be helped to understand the range of feelings they may experience, that they are normal and that they will change over time.

The words a carer uses at that time may well be remembered. A parent who has just lost a child, or knows they will lose that child, is very sensitive to someone projecting their own feelings or to feeling unheard; but they can be reassured and comforted by empathetic listening. They may be feeling guilt, shame or anger, as well as the pain, and will look for those feelings to be mirrored in those around them. Hearing that those feelings are normal and knowing someone else has felt a little like that can help to relieve some of the sense of isolation.

> *Jackie attended for her 20-week scan, very excited at the thought of seeing her baby and hopefully learning its gender. She already had a 4-year-old son and she and her partner were hoping this would be a girl to complete their family.*
>
> *Jackie noticed that the sonographer seemed to be taking his time with the scan. Then he slowly turned to her and said that sadly, the baby had not grown past 16 weeks and there was no heartbeat. Jackie was understandably shocked. She became angry with the sonographer, shouting at him that he must be wrong and demanding that someone else check. Checking the findings of the scan is normal practice if a death is suspected*

*and so another sonographer quickly arrived. He sadly confirmed the diagnosis. Throughout the next steps, Jackie appeared very anxious and required a great deal of support from both her partner and the team dealing with her.*

*Jackie did not know that this was the first time the sonographer had scanned a baby death and had to tell a mother that her baby had died. He was very shocked by Jackie's anger. He went home early that day then phoned in sick the next morning. When he returned to work, the colleague who had confirmed the death with him was able to share some of her experiences; help him review his communication with Jackie; and to better understand anger and its relation to loss. He was then encouraged to consider what had affected him about the anger displayed, which led him to reflect on some personal issues relating to anger. It was important for him to develop a professional response to anger in which he could separate his personal feelings from a considered, professional approach.*

## THE GRIEVING PROCESS

Grief is frightening and disturbing. It can bring unexpected symptoms such as anger and the 'pangs' of grief that seem to come from nowhere. Some people may also experience physical illness related to the loss.

We are all affected in the way we grieve by our culture: our national culture, our religious culture and the culture of our family. It is important not to make assumptions based on our own culture about how others will deal with grief. Some may believe that the death was at the will of their god and that to go against this with prolonged grieving would be inappropriate or disrespectful. For some, death is a part of life and accepted as such. Others are supported by the rituals and norms of their religious or family culture and grandparents and other family members can be included in the grieving. We must always check with a family as to what is helpful and important to them.

Rituals surrounding death and mourning are among humanity's few truly universal practices. All societies have some form of funeral ceremony. The purpose of this as described by Bowlby[1] is threefold: to help the bereaved to recognise and make real the loss; to take note publicly of the loss; to provide a focus for the community; and to ensure "the lost one continues the relationship with the living". Cultures vary in how they deal with, acknowledge and honour loss. The commonly felt anger may also be contained by these rituals. Uncontained, it can be turned on the self or others.

There are several models of grieving that may be helpful to people supporting those experiencing a loss. Sometimes, just knowing that the way you are feeling is normal and will pass can be a huge relief. This may be all a busy professional can do at times but many of those who have suffered a loss have found it invaluable. Grief can feel very lonely and to know there is someone who understands you need time and permission to grieve can really make a difference.

## THE PROCESS OF MOURNING

Several well-known mental health writers have described the tasks of mourning. In the 1960s and 70s, Elizabeth Kubler Ross[2] explored five stages of grief: denial, anger, bargaining, depression and acceptance. Using four-stage models, John Bowlby[3] in the 1970s and 1980s and Colin Murray-Parkes[4] at around the same time, explored the stages and effects of grief and their resolution.

Their work has given a lasting basis for understanding the process of mourning. More recently, practitioners have been less fixed in how mourning is regarded but those four tasks still give us a useful way of looking at what to expect and how to help people move through loss to acceptance.

Engel[5] sees the process of mourning as healing. He compares it to a skin cut: a small graze will gradually heal by itself but a deep cut needs attention, or it will never properly heal and will leave a scar. We need time and support to bring a body back into balance. It is a normal and healthy process. Grief after loss disturbs the physiology of the human body and the process of mourning is necessary to restore it. Some people feel actual physical pain and the mourning process can be clouded by attention to physical symptoms at the expense of psychological ones.

*Each day on the postnatal ward, Jenny came up with different physical symptoms. She had been through a long and difficult labour and, because she had haemorrhaged after delivery, she had been admitted to ITU for two days. The staff were understandably anxious about her physical recovery. Her partner had been very involved in caring for their newborn. This gave him a role in what had been a frightening experience for him. None of the symptoms uncovered further complications and Jenny was allowed home.*

*The community midwife visiting her raised the subject of Jenny's recurrent fears about her health and she broke down in tears and sobbed. Whilst to a counsellor this would seem entirely appropriate, the midwife felt a little at a loss to know how to help her. Should she be able to manage this situation? What would help her client? Returning to Jenny with an offer of counselling helped the midwife to feel she had opened the door for her to receive the help she needed to start to deal with her feelings; although she couldn't control the fact that Jenny took some time to respond.*

*When Jenny attended the first session, she was very worried about her uncontrollable tears and the frightening feelings she was experiencing. She tried to put them to the back of her mind but at unexpected moments she would dissolve in tears and feel panicky. She had also experienced flashbacks to her emergency situation after the delivery. All this left her feeling very anxious. Her family told her how ill she had been and how lucky she was to be alive, starkly reminding her that her life had been in danger. It took several sessions talking step-by-step through what had actually happened during Jenny's labour for her to feel a little more settled and that what had happened was in the past.*

*What Jenny had 'lost' was the first precious days with her baby and her faith in her health. She wanted to regain some control of her life by understanding step by step the processes that had led to the emergency and the care she was given. She was then able to put in place the mechanisms she needed to manage and to feel in control again. Jenny also felt her husband would benefit from having a session with the counsellor where he could talk through his feelings around this traumatic experience.*

*They subsequently all met together with the baby and Jenny and her husband were able to share with each other what would help them recover and how they could best support one another and look forward to being happy with her baby.*

It may be helpful for those who are bereaved to first understand the mourning process they need to experience in order to recover. Just as in the models of grieving, no-one mourns in the same way as someone else. There are, however, common features that many will experience. Psychologists do not all agree on the order of the stages, nor even that they all occur, but they may be a useful guideline. Worden[6] suggested four tasks of mourning:

- Acceptance
- Experience of the pain
- Adjusting to a new environment
- Finding an enduring connection with the lost one while embarking on a new life

## CULTURAL DIFFERENCES IN MOURNING

There are cultural differences in how loss and mourning are regarded and experienced. In some societies, people are often protected from the reality of loss until they themselves experience it, leaving them confused and overwhelmed. In some, there is an acceptance and expectation of very open mourning and public distress. In others, it's the rituals around loss which are important and must be observed.

It may be appropriate if you are unsure to ask your client if they have any expectations of how they want to manage the situation. Some people will not want others involved, whilst some may embrace the support and shared grieving of the whole family or wider community.

> *Sajeeta and Dipesh were 37 weeks pregnant when she was told that their baby had died in the womb. Sajeeta's command of English was poor but Dipesh was quite fluent. After the shock, and when the couple appeared ready for an explanation of the process for labour and delivery using an interpreter, Dipesh asked the midwife if he could have a private word. He asked her to take the baby away immediately at birth and not to let his wife see it. This gave the midwife caring for Sajeeta a dilemma. It is usual when working with the labouring woman to establish her wishes for the management of that precious time with her baby. In order to understand the differing needs of each couple, sometimes more knowledge is required.*

> *Talking to the family about their customs around death helps the midwife to deliver care appropriately and in this situation the midwife felt she should check what Sajeeta wanted with the interpreter.*

It is important not to fear not knowing the customs or rituals of another culture or religion. Asking sensitively and admitting to not knowing will not generally offend and the wish to be helpful and supportive will often overcome the client having to explain. Indeed, sometimes the explanation will help them to be clear about what matters to them. Help can also be found from hospital chaplains and local faith leaders, who will have contacts and can guide anyone who is unsure about observances.

# CULTURAL DIFFERENCES FOR PROFESSIONALS

Using the information detailed above enables the professional to remain focused on the needs of the family but this may challenge the professionals' personal beliefs. Positively, this can lead to an increased appreciation of and sensitivity towards cultural issues and cross-cultural care. It can also lead to some confusion and deserves support to enable an understanding of how and why these differences can be managed in order to maintain the professional relationship. Support may be found by talking to community members, or to colleagues and friends with experience of managing similar issues.

# SIBLINGS AND LOSS

Whilst the parents and the professionals may be given attention, it is also helpful if siblings have had a chance to hear about and perhaps meet the baby. Most will have known a baby was coming and they need to know what has happened. They may well observe parents' distress or overhear conversations.

Depending on their age, children may not be able to understand but they will need reassurance, particularly that it is not their fault. Young children are the centre of their own world and often believe they affect all that happens around them. Younger children may not have any concept of the permanence of death.

Children over about 6 years may understand and accept more. It is important that parents recognise they sometimes may not display any emotions, but these may well emerge in behaviours, play or sometimes, disturbed sleep. These things are normal and will generally pass. It may help if the parents are able to speak about the lost baby to them in as positive a way as they can manage.

Dealing with denial can be difficult. It helps if a parent has had time with the dead child and has felt that connection to them. This is not always possible, and the parents will sometimes need to process their feelings without that. Honesty and clear information about what happened to the baby, even if that means saying, "I don't know", helps to reassure them that they are not responsible.

# RELATIONSHIPS WITH PROFESSIONALS

Reassurance from the professionals that everything was done to try to save the baby may be questioned but it does help parents to accept and trust the professionals. Longer-term denial is likely to lead to problems in re-establishing a healthy life and good relationships; and could resurface with a subsequent pregnancy. Present grief will often bring back past losses not given sufficient reflection at the time.

Clients may need professional support to manage such feelings. Whilst most midwives will not need to deal with these in depth, it may be helpful to recognise them and how they could be impeding the client's relationship to the present pregnancy. This is described as Dependent Grief, when the bereaved person is still clinging emotionally to the lost one; Unexpected Loss syndrome, when the shock and denial become an anxiety state; and Conflicted Grief syndrome when an ambivalent relationship with the lost one may perpetuate the grieving and delay resolution.

*The GP asked the bereavement midwife to contact Sheri as she had been to the surgery quite a few times after the loss of her baby and he was concerned about her mental health. Sheri agreed to meet the midwife but did not want to come to the hospital as it brought back too many memories.*

*On the first home visit, the midwife was a little taken aback by the number of photographs of her lost baby around the living room. Sheri said it helped her to have them as she felt close to her little one with them there. She said that she had been angry with her partner when he suggested she should take some of them down. Her sister had been shocked when she visited her and said she would not come again as she found it too painful to see all the photos.*

*During this first session, Sheri was challenged to look further into her reasons for the display of photographs. The emerging theme seemed to the midwife to be that of wanting to hold on to her loss and she explored this with Sheri. Sheri feared that if she took the photos down, others would think that she was no longer feeling sad most of the time and they would want her to be "better". Surrounded by her baby photos, she felt comforted. If her baby had been alive, of course she would be with her all the time and this would be normal and expected, so maybe this was another factor in the loss Sheri was experiencing.*

*Listening to Sheri explain what this loss meant to her, talking about the baby and what she had felt whilst in mourning for her, was really important. Sheri's visits to her doctor had been her cry for help in the middle of all these confusing feelings.*

## THE END OF MOURNING

For some people the shock of the loss and its effects on their lives, hopes and plans, means they feel they may never stop grieving, or that it would be wrong to stop, as that would feel like a betrayal of the lost one. Helping the bereaved to see that there can be a normal process of grieving and that they need time and support to reach a place where they can feel whole, can be invaluable. It may not always come at the right time, but any support *will* have an effect.

There may also be unconscious limits on grief. People who have suffered a loss may feel that they have to be 'over it' in a certain time and that to grieve for longer is unacceptable or a sign of mental ill health. They may find those around them are supportive and sympathetic for a period but then begin to drift away or to suggest they should be getting over it. Some cultures deal with the loss and grieving quickly and soon feel that it no longer needs to be acknowledged. There is no timescale for grieving, and it is important that the bereaved are reassured on this. It may be that for some, the grieving will not end, and they will need help to manage that. Many parents in a bereavement group run by analyst Judith Savage[7] vowed "never to forget" their lost child and were most distressed when they felt that others had forgotten. They felt that their identity as parents had been unacknowledged, yet for them this was still felt as their reality.

*Greta came back to see the counsellor following the loss of her baby at 18 weeks. This had happened 2 months ago. Her husband was worried that she was, "not getting over" her loss. He felt she should be back to what he perceived as normal. Greta sobbed as she sat in the counselling room. She had not yet found the words to explain her feelings about her loss. Slowly, as we talked about her baby and what she had expected during her pregnancy, the words of loss began to form as she expressed her disbelief, sadness, anger; and she cried.*

*Working with her feelings enabled her to let them out and receive the validation that these were appropriate for her grief. Her husband found sitting through this difficult. His felt his role was to try to protect her from the pain. His anxiety about her mental health was eased by helping him to understand that being alongside her and allowing her to grieve was the best support he could give.*

Often in these situations, professionals, midwives and GPs can feel intimidated, uncertain and at a loss as to how to help. Recognising this pattern and explaining how change can happen helps the couple to manage their grief. There are no rights or wrongs and no time restrictions. We will only move forward at our own pace when we have the support we need. People need to understand that there may always be lingering painful feelings around the loss and that finding ways to manage those is important for the future.

Those who have lost someone close need to be given permission to do whatever helps them. That may be to cry or to shout or to sit quiet and still. Those supporting them at this time can help a great deal just by accepting the need to express the painful feelings, which can be extreme and frightening for the client. Some people may deny the loss or the need to grieve and this, too, is a coping mechanism which they will need help to manage and from which to move to an acknowledgment of the loss. We must not assume that everyone who experiences a loss will be traumatized. Most will grieve in their own way and feel some ending. It is thought that only 5-10% experience PTSD (Post Traumatic Stress Disorder).

Our greatest attachment is usually to our children or future children. The pain of loss is related to our attachment. Separation from an attachment figure causes fear and anxiety; permanent separation pain and grief, and sometimes later difficulties in adjusting and forming new attachments. There is no 'proper' way to grieve and there are no rules for grieving, but we do know that talking about the loss, making it real, acknowledging the experience and the lost expectations, all help to prevent depression arising later.

It is sometimes difficult for couples who have lost a child at any stage to recognise that they may be grieving in different ways.

*Rose and Alan lost a baby to stillbirth. They went home immediately from the hospital, feeling they did not need to talk to anyone as they both had parents nearby who they thought would help them. Rose's mother had experienced a miscarriage many years before. She had not had anyone to talk to and had suffered from depression in later life, so she encouraged Rose to talk about the baby and to cry when she needed to. Rose says that she cried non-stop for weeks but that she was allowed to do it and she felt "silly but relieved". Alan's parents were on the phone, anxious to help, but Rose felt they didn't really want to talk.*

*Alan felt he had "no excuse" to stay off work and went back the next day. He found it impossible to talk about the loss and said later that his friends and colleagues were "relieved" that he did not want to engage them with his feelings. Alan felt he needed to protect Rose from how he was feeling, so he tried to hide it.*

*Rose began to feel that Alan was not grieving and had not really cared about the baby. She found it too hard to bring this up, as she would just burst into tears again and she wanted to protect her husband. However, she felt increasingly angry and distant.*

*It was only when they decided to try for another baby that the distance between them became clear and they decided to seek help. If they had understood earlier the value of talking about feelings even though it is difficult and painful, they may have avoided two years of distance and anger.*

## INVESTING IN ANOTHER RELATIONSHIP

Acceptance is the first step, but it may not come immediately. There is often a period of numbness immediately after a loss which allows people to deal with the 'business' of loss: the administrative tasks and the plans for a funeral. After the numbness may be a denial of the reality of the loss and anger at what has happened. This may be directed at the lost one, at themselves or those around them who did not stop this from happening. This phase of "yearning", as Worden describes it, begins to accept the reality while longing for the lost one.

The next phase may be one of disorganisation, of finding it difficult to cope with everyday life, gradually moving towards reorganisation and managing life without the daily pain and anger. Investing in another relationship is often the phase of mourning at which health professionals become involved. A new pregnancy is a source of joy, but the inevitable anxiety is another step on the path of mourning. If women and their partners are aware of this, it may help them to be less fearful.

These phases are not experienced by everyone or even in this order, but it may be useful for the professional to have them in mind, and to accept the feelings and fears of each stage of experience. They may be particularly affected by the anger directed at the lost one or at those felt to be responsible for the loss. The later anxiety (and sometimes anger) at investing in a new relationship can also be mitigated by the health professionals who encounter it and can reassure clients that this, too, is a part of mourning.

# 2: The First Trimester: Conception to 12 Weeks

*The secret weeks; early pregnancy loss; early pregnancy loss (miscarriage); early pregnancy loss (termination); talking about loss; first contact with the professionals; talking about uncertainty: ectopic pregnancy and molar pregnancy; longer-term effects of early loss; information and support.*

Reactions to a positive pregnancy test may be unexpected, both to the pregnant woman and to those around her. She may have planned the pregnancy but find she has doubts when it becomes real; or may have to deal with other people's negative reactions. The huge change that pregnancy brings may make some women joyful and glowing with positive anticipation but for others, it will become a fearful time and they may feel this is wrong and too difficult to discuss.

If professionals do not have expectations about how a client will react, it will help them to feel able to explore their feelings without fear of judgement. How we make decisions, where we find our information and how we evaluate it are all affected by the emotional reaction to a pregnancy. These decisions often have to be made quickly and knowing there is help and support will enable women and their partners to move forward.

## THE SECRET WEEKS: WHO TO TELL AND WHAT TO TELL

There are difficulties, anxieties and losses that can occur at all stages of pregnancy, before pregnancy and after delivery that may require help and support. Each period has particular areas that challenge both the client and the professionals. We have referred to the early weeks as the 'secret weeks' because it is a time when many women and couples are not ready to talk about the pregnancy. This may be because they want to be sure that all is well before announcing it, or they may be uncertain whether they want to continue the pregnancy, or about who should know. Once the pregnancy has been disclosed to anyone, a decision has been made and others will have to follow. In the early weeks, these decisions can cause anxiety and uncertainty for many parents.

These are some of the challenges that the professionals are going to face in talking to parents about their choices and the future, as well as about how to manage the present. These are not actions that can be changed once a decision is made and this can feel paralysing for clients without information and support.

Pregnancy loss after assisted conception may carry its own particular pain. It may be that the method of conception has not been made known or there may be some fear of stigma, particularly if a termination is sought.

## EARLY PREGNANCY LOSS

Early pregnancy loss, whether through miscarriage, termination or an early diagnosis of foetal abnormality, can result in grief that may be felt as anger, sadness, deep distress or despair, when people feel hopeless and helpless and their difficulty in coping can lead to withdrawal and/or depression. It changes their view of the future and how they may feel about a subsequent pregnancy. It affects both partners, although they may respond differently. In some cultures, there are different expectations of how a woman should respond to and deal with such a loss. The expectations on men in relation to loss also vary with culture, religion and family mores; and can be very powerful in affecting male identity.

Early loss not only affects the woman and her partner, if he or she is involved, but also sometimes her family, friends, co-workers, and the medical professionals who may be involved at all stages of the pregnancy and loss. They will all bring their own experiences, expectations and prejudices to their response to the event. Annemarie Jutel[1] argues that, "we must make pregnant women's attitudes central and focus on whether or not a pregnant woman regards the loss of the pregnancy as the loss of a child". This gives us a guide as to how to communicate with that woman, and not to assume that all women will feel the same way.

Men involved with early pregnancy loss may not react as expected by their partner or by medical professionals. McCreight[2] in her study of male participants in a support group, found that some fathers felt under pressure not to express their grief, either to conform to a masculine identity or because they felt that this would support their partner. Where the life partner is a woman, they will often also grieve the loss but may feel that their feelings are not acknowledged or addressed. Peel & Ellis[3].

## MISCARRIAGE

Many health professionals have little experience of early pregnancy loss. It may not even come to the attention of a GP, despite the frequency of such losses. It is estimated that 30-40% of conceptions do not end in a live birth. Figures from the USA suggest that 25% of women will experience an early pregnancy loss (Trends in Pregnancy Loss among US women 1990-2011-2017).

It is sometimes assumed there will be no grieving for a baby that was "hardly there" and psychological sequelae may be ignored. If staff expect there may be emotional distress after the loss, they are more likely to detect and assess it, and to give the woman the space and listening that she may need. Grieving may not happen immediately when people are numb or trying to process what has happened to them. They may seem to be coping or feel that they must be seen to be coping when they have made the decision themselves, leaving those close to them relieved and paying less attention. The signs of grief - tearfulness, anger, low mood and guilt - may come later and may not even be associated with the loss.

*Alice was a 29-year-old office worker with a daughter of eighteen months. She had recently returned to work part-time while her mother cared for Jenny two days a week and she spent one day in a workplace nursery. Alice and her partner had been delighted to be pregnant again as they wanted the children close in age. She had started to make plans for her maternity leave and the care for Jenny. At ten weeks, Alice miscarried the baby.*

*She saw her GP, who was kind but did not offer any support or show empathy with how she might feel. Alice returned to work immediately, tried to forget about it and try again.*

*After about two months, she began to feel lacking in energy and motivation. She no longer enjoyed her days with Jenny and would ask her mother to have her an extra day. She felt there may be something physically wrong, so the GP did blood tests and pressure checks. There was nothing obvious but her family and then a health visitor friend grew concerned. She did not want to discuss her feelings with them and became angry if they encouraged her.*

*After a few weeks, her friend raised the subject of the miscarriage and wondered if that might have had more effect on her than Alice had believed. At first, she blamed not getting pregnant again for her mood, but then agreed that she had never really grieved for the lost baby, even though she had been so excited and had made preparations.*

*She took time to accept that she could mourn the baby and that it had been a real part of her life and grief was normal. She had felt that because it was "not a real baby yet" that it was not appropriate to experience the loss. Alice found it difficult to allow herself to be sad and angry and to recognise that those feelings were normal and would pass. She had begun to feel better by the time she was pregnant again, but found the pregnancy made her very anxious and she needed more support and time to feel safe again. Helping her talk about the loss and what it had meant to the whole family meant that Alice could allow herself to feel that the baby had been "real", and the loss had entirely normal effects on her. It did not mean that she was "mad or bad" as she had begun to think.*

For some women and their partners, miscarriage is felt as a bereavement and for them it should be validated as such. Not all women feel that way, but for everyone it is a transitional, complex event.

Organisations such as the Miscarriage Association provide information and support for women who are in danger of losing or who have lost a baby by miscarriage; as well as for professionals who want more information. Sharing their stories and feelings helps many people, both men and women, to feel less lonely within their experience.

Women who lose a pregnancy in the very early weeks may have no opportunity to talk about their feelings of loss. It was long considered by the medical professions to be of little importance and many pregnancies ended without the mother being aware that she was pregnant. Information using pregnancy apps and modern technology has resulted in more women being aware of and relating to the pregnancy in the early weeks, but they are not always moderated by professionals and so the information they convey cannot always be relied upon to be medically correct. Women may not be followed up medically after a miscarriage, even if they have been admitted to a hospital, and so the impact of early loss may not be recognised by doctors or midwives. because it is outside of their experience. However, many women and men do feel the loss hugely. They have 'felt pregnant' as soon as they knew and have almost always started to make plans for their future with their child. Losing the baby means that the future they saw for themselves, whether this is a first or subsequent pregnancy, has to be rewritten.

It is difficult to predict who will suffer the most common emotional disorders – depression and anxiety - after a miscarriage. A study in the British Journal of Psychiatry by Blackmore[4] showed a higher risk of depression postpartum in those who had suffered miscarriage. Of 2,823 women in the study who had suffered miscarriages, around 15% had experienced clinically significant depression and/or anxiety during and after further pregnancies for three years. Just who will be affected depends on many factors, including the woman's past mental health, the level of support she has and her coping strategies. The stage of loss she is at does not seem to be significant in the level of grief, depression or anxiety.

## TERMINATION

The English Abortion Act 1967 allows legal termination of pregnancy up to 24 weeks with the agreement of two medical practitioners acting in good faith. The grounds for termination as stated in the Act are that the continuation of the pregnancy would cause injury to the physical or mental health of the mother or any existing children; or that the continuance of the pregnancy would put the life of the woman at risk; or that there is a risk that if the child were born it would suffer serious physical or mental handicap. This has applied ever since in the United Kingdom, and in Northern Ireland from October 2019, when abortion was decriminalised. Debates continue about what "good faith" means, and the meaning of "handicap" or "risk to health" The BPAS (British Pregnancy Advisory Service) website has a series of informative articles on many of these matters.

Terminating a pregnancy is affected by religious, cultural and political views. Traditional views on termination were foetus-centric, involving the rights of the child and the moral value of life. This has resulted in the polarising debate over whether or not, in the early weeks, a foetus is a human being. This focus has shifted in some parts of the world in more recent times to encompass the feelings of the woman and the outcome of the loss on her mental state. There are still countries that do not give women the right to decide to end a pregnancy in the first few weeks.

Guillaume and Rossier[5] offer an overview of international legislation and measures on abortion. Lindemann[6] describes the "calling into personhood" of the foetus as a turning point in how women regard their pregnancy. Many pregnant women do this as soon as they have the pregnancy confirmed: 'This is a child and I am a mother'; others do not, or do not want to consider the 'humanness' of the foetus. This may shape and be shaped by how they regard the pregnancy and themselves.

In their social world, if they have told people about the pregnancy, that may also begin to change their perceptions of self and so even a chosen loss at this time means the loss of the child and the loss of the role of parent.

Women choose to have a termination for many reasons. They may feel that they do not have support financially or socially or it may be for health reasons. Some women did not want to be pregnant and do not want to consider continuing the pregnancy. The pregnancy may be as a result of abuse or rape. Some may have wanted to be pregnant, but the reality may have changed their feelings; or the reactions of others - perhaps the withdrawal of support - may have led them to feel that they would not be able to cope. Some women may have to make decisions about continuing a pregnancy with a foetal abnormality; and others with ectopic or molar pregnancies will not have the choice.

We must not assume that all women who experience a pregnancy loss will respond the same way. Some seek out help and support[7], whilst others may feel they have adequate coping strategies or support within their communities. There are some who cope by denying it and may find future pregnancies more challenging.

However common and seemingly acceptable early termination by choice has become, there are about 200,000 performed in England and Wales each year (Department of Health and Social Care), it still has negative effects on a number of women. Even in European countries with the unconditional right to terminate before 12 weeks, emotional distress following termination is quite common.

Studies in this area are of necessity qualitative, as it is not possible to randomise a study of termination. This means that they may not be generalised to the population, but they do give some insight into the negative and positive effects of termination.

A review of studies by Allyson Lipp[8] showed some negative impacts of termination in the first trimester, revealing some indicators for negative psychological consequences. In a Norwegian study following up on this after two years, Broen et al[9] found that pressure from a male partner to terminate a pregnancy was the strongest predictor of emotional distress.

Other studies, such as Cozzarelli in the US[10], found that those women with low self-esteem were least likely to find help and support, particularly from partners, and felt less able to manage negative feelings. In a long-term overview in Australia, Bonevski and Adams[11] found that negative psychological outcomes were found most in women with prior mental illness, low self-esteem, late gestation termination and those conflicted by religious or cultural beliefs. From a range of studies, Lipp[8] found that prior mental illness is likely to indicate a need for greater support. This includes a history of self-harm, depression and suicide in the family, as well as illnesses such as schizophrenia and bipolar disorder.

It is important that professionals dealing with early pregnancy termination are aware of the possible psychological effects and of the indicators for negative responses. Zolese & Blacker[12] found that 10% of women showed some disturbance, mainly anxiety and depression. Bonevski and Adams[11] found no difference in levels of distress in the type of procedure, or in teenagers as compared to older women. The raised levels of grief were found most amongst those undergoing termination for foetal abnormality.

The way women cope with the psychological effects of termination varies with their previous experiences, the level of support they have and their expectations. Different studies have found the effects of coping strategies such as making the foetus a person, have both negative and positive effects. This may be because other issues are affecting the woman that make it hard for her to process the feelings, deal with the memories and release the guilt.

We should be aware that not all women who terminate a pregnancy have negative outcomes. A large study by Gilchrist et al[13] found that when previous psychiatric history was controlled for psychiatric disorders, emotional problems were no higher following termination than following childbirth. Some may think that if a woman has chosen to end the pregnancy there will only be relief and, whilst that may be part of her response, research shows that some women do experience doubt, guilt and grieving. The reasons behind choosing to terminate a pregnancy are many and will affect the woman's responses to it. They will also be affected by how other people in their social world respond and whether they feel judged or supported. The women who had the most support from a partner showed the fewest negative responses Broen[9].

We can see from some of the research that women who are in conflict with their religious beliefs or the norms of their culture in seeking or agreeing to termination are more likely to suffer negative psychological outcomes. An Irish review by Clare & Tyrrell[14] showed that religious conflict was a determinant of negative psychological outcomes. It may be very important for these women to have access to support throughout and after the termination from someone who will help them to explore and confront the conflicts they may experience.

Midwives may also have an opportunity to explore some of these feelings when women have future pregnancies, although not all will disclose a previous termination.

## TERMINATION AND THE PROFESSIONAL

Attitudes to termination have changed over the last few decades, but clients may still be unsure about the reaction they will receive from the professionals and how to present themselves. Some women attending a termination service are very unsure about how to talk to the staff. They feel they must be certain in wanting a termination and that to express any concern or uncertainty means they will be refused. They do not always feel able to tell the truth to a complete stranger, particularly as it may involve underage sex, incest, abuse or being under threat. It can be very difficult for staff in a TOP (Termination of Pregnancy) clinic to assess in a short time the situation a client may be in, even if they can sense there may be a problem. It may only be possible to offer a chance to express their feelings and fears in an open way. The issue of confidentiality may be difficult in this area, particularly if the client is underage or reports abuse. They may ask that the information is not shared with anyone else, but the health professional may need to act on it. This must be made clear to the client even if it changes the relationship with them.

Safeguarding may be an issue with young pregnant women, particularly if they do not want parents or guardians to be told. At 16 years old, young people are considered competent to make a decision about termination. Below this age, they need to demonstrate sufficient understanding and maturity. They may be judged by the Gillick or Fraser guidelines. These were introduced in the UK to assess a young person's competence to be given contraception without parental consent but may also be applied to termination.

The young person may need to be offered extra support or counselling. although staff must be prepared for them to reject this, perhaps out fear or from being unfamiliar with discussing their feelings. Whilst there may be an awareness by staff that a young woman's pregnancy may be an indicator of exploitation, it is only by giving them space and a non-judgmental approach that she may be able to let anyone know the situation. Giving out contact numbers or email contacts may mean that some will feel able to make contact for support after a termination.

Some of the staff caring for women in pregnancy may have objections to terminations and this must be respected by managers and colleagues. However, it is important that staff do not convey their own feelings to the woman concerned either, negatively or positively. The woman must make the decision and feel supported in doing so, whatever that decision may be. Medical professionals may also have negative or positive feelings about termination arising from their own direct experience, or that of someone close. As we will discuss in a later chapter, being aware of our own feelings and prejudices helps us to put them aside and to focus on the needs of the client.

The RCN publishes guidelines on abortion care which cover all areas of practice for nurses and midwives.

## RESEARCH ON TERMINATION IN THE FIRST TRIMESTER: PSYCHOLOGICAL EFFECTS

The available research on the psychological effects of first trimester termination generally shows that women who have chosen to end a pregnancy do not experience a bad outcome. A review of the literature by Fine-Davis,[15] published in 2007 concludes that, "legal and voluntary termination of pregnancy rarely causes immediate or lasting negative psychological consequences in healthy women". They found that when negative psychological effects did occur, they were mainly "mild and transient", and these were seen within the normal framework of stress and coping.

Stotland[16] concluded that postpartum women were eight times more likely to have negative psychological outcomes than those having a voluntary first trimester termination. For first trimester terminations, most studies found that the women were most likely to experience relief. There are some exceptions and women who have a history of mental ill health are more likely to have further problems after termination. This may also apply to women whose religious beliefs preclude abortion Clare and Tyrrell[14].

Feelings of regret were more often expressed by women who had a strong relationship with their partner[17]. This was associated with sadness rather than negative psychological outcomes. Whilst this research is over thirty years old and attitudes have changed over the intervening years, it still has some value in an area where there is little research.

## TALKING ABOUT LOSS

*Joy attended a pregnancy advice centre saying she had done a pregnancy test with a positive result and she did not know what to do. She explained her situation: an on/off boyfriend and a new job, shared accommodation and a relationship with her mother that she described as "ok, but not close". She found it very difficult to discuss her feelings about the pregnancy but said that talking about it made it "real" and forced her to realise she would have to make the decision. She did not expect support from anyone and expected her family would judge her and that she would "fail again", this time as a mother.*

*It seemed that Joy was unsure about what being a mother would mean for her and that this would be a good area to help her to explore. For many women, the uncertainty about the mothering role, particularly if their own experience of being mothered is not a good one, may make them doubtful about their own ability to mother. Joy's use of the word "fail" seemed pertinent: where she felt she had failed and what failure means to her. Reflecting back her own words as "you said that you felt you would fail?" and leaving space for her to respond made it seem less judgmental and allowed her to develop what she was trying to express.*

In the early weeks, women have to decide who they will tell about the pregnancy. For someone who is delighted and feels she has support and people to share it with who will be positive about it, there may not be any hesitation. For those who are not sure whether they want to be pregnant, or if they will have any support, or expecting a negative and possibly life-changing reaction to the news, there will be huge questions about who to tell and when. Some women are so unsure that they go into a state of denial and blank out the pregnancy. Others try to hide it for as long as possible and will appear very late, if at all, at antenatal services. Their reasons may depend on their previous experience or their expectations of support or fear of judgement. The reactions of the first people told may affect the decisions they make.

*Cerys was very reluctant to attend a booking appointment. She had seen her GP but did not want to answer questions or discuss her plans. She was referred to the counsellor as the GP was concerned that if she wanted a termination, the time was running out and the GP wanted her to see the midwife. The note from the doctor said that Cerys was 19 years old but that she knew very little about her, as she had rarely attended the surgery. She had told the GP that she had recently returned to live with her single mother but would not say any more.*

*At her first appointment she was very tense and looked at the ground. She started to answer some unthreatening questions about herself but then stopped and said that this was why she did not want to see the midwife because she knew that she would "ask too many questions and decide what I'm like and what I need. I can look things up on the internet if I need to know them". It seemed that for Cerys, support and interrogation were one and the same. It was important to acknowledge that she had things she did not want to talk about, and that was fine; but they did need to think about some things that were crucial for her and the baby.*

*Asking Cerys to talk about herself in a non-judgmental way in fairly general terms helped her to feel less that she was being asked lots of questions. "Tell me a bit about yourself" often elicits more information and seems less threatening. Making it clear that you are listening to the story helps the client to sense your empathy.*

Women may be uncertain what they should tell the professionals they meet. Everyone edits what they say at some level and anxiety about the questions you may be asked or how someone will react to your answers affects what you choose to say. Many people feel they need to be "a good patient" and that will mean they will not necessarily feel free to be honest about or even know what they are feeling. They may feel regret or shame about their past experiences, leaving them reluctant to open up to a stranger.

Open questions and an empathetic manner may help them to gradually accept that the professionals are on their side and will not make judgements. Some women may be reluctant to talk about previous pregnancies, especially if they have had terminations, and more so if their partners or family know nothing about this. They may also be unsure about letting people know that this is a donor pregnancy or that the father's identity is uncertain. Whether or not to tell the truth is a decision about how that truth will be received, how much confidentiality can be trusted and how you feel after a secret has been revealed.

*Sangita was a 27-year-old woman of Indian origin, from what she described as a "very traditional family". She had been married for two years and was working as a teacher in an inner-city school. She had answered all the midwife's questions but seemed reluctant to engage in any conversation. The GP had written that this was a first pregnancy and the couple were very positive about it.*

*The midwife was concerned that Sangita did not seem very positive. In fact, she felt that Sangita was anxious to finish and leave as soon as possible. She checked with Sangita that this was her first pregnancy. Sangita burst into tears and said that she wanted to leave. The midwife tried to calm her but felt she needed to understand what was happening even with the time pressure she was under. Sangita eventually said that she had had a termination whilst at university but neither her husband nor any of her family knew and they would, "all hate me for it".*

*It clearly helped Sangita to talk briefly about the circumstances of the termination. She was still bearing some of the burden of that decision. Her comment that the family "would hate her" may in fact be a projection of how she felt about herself. Being able to express and examine her reasons for that difficult decision helped her to better deal with the current pregnancy.*

Sometimes women forget the very good reasons that they had at the time for a termination. Their social or financial situations, the circumstances of the conception or just the fear of the future. Although there is much research that says there are few long-term psychological effects of termination, some women do continue to feel guilt and sometimes, regret. Regret is not a psychological condition, but it can be burdensome. Some women continue to feel anxious or depressed after a termination, sometimes for years afterwards; and a new pregnancy can bring back these feelings. Helping them to remember the fear, panic or aloneness some felt may help them to recognise the reasons they made that choice, and to be a little less hard on themselves.

## TALKING ABOUT UNCERTAINTY: THE FIRST CONTACTS WITH PROFESSIONALS

A pregnancy changes all the relationships you have. A single woman or a couple are now a family and parents are grandparents. Single, childless friends and relatives may feel that they will be less important, or that you will not be so available. Even colleagues will sense a change of focus and may fear that your work will be affected. Partners, even supportive ones, notice differences. Not everyone is prepared for this change in relationships and it can cause anxiety and even anger. The woman may feel that she is still exactly the same person but that everyone is treating her differently. Cultural aspects and religious aspects of parenthood all begin to be felt.

*Jessie was seen at home following her miscarriage. Both of the sisters she lived with were pregnant and this was causing her much distress. They had shared every pregnancy detail and experience and now she felt very alone with her loss. It also seemed to her that her sisters and their partners were avoiding her and were not at all interested in discussing her needs. She felt anxious in the house and was becoming very angry at her family. Her own boyfriend walked away when she cried. Having someone to acknowledge her loss and offer her time and space to experience all her feelings about it gave her the time to let go of her pain and some of her anger.*

*The sessions also enabled Jessie to work out what she wanted and needed from her partner and family, to face them and have open discussions about her feelings. This in turn allowed them to recognize what this loss had meant for each of them individually, because all the family were affected. The sisters also felt encouraged to open up and talk to their midwives and share their own worries and fears.*

Expectations of yourself, your partner, your family and the larger group around you will be affected by your previous experiences and the society in which you grew up. How everyone copes with a pregnancy/new baby/more children will depend on the woman's (and in some cases, the family's) social, financial and cultural circumstances. Some families and some cultures will welcome a new addition, whatever the circumstances, and will find a way to manage. Other women may find themselves isolated and struggling to cope. They may feel ashamed to talk about this and will need support and an open questioning to help them.

*Kara attended the first appointment with her mother. Her mother seemed to be answering all the questions and Kara said little, even when addressed directly. The midwife wanted to ask her mother to leave but when she started to suggest it, Kara was distressed and said her mother wanted to be involved and that was fine. It emerged that Kara had two children of five and two years who were cared for by her mother whilst Kara worked. Her mother seemed quite hostile during the session and the midwife was uncertain about Kara's feelings. Finding a space for Kara was important or no one would know how she was feeling about the pregnancy of which it seems her mother had taken possession.*

*Kara needed to have time to speak, so the midwife suggested that she had to do a physical examination with her alone. This seemed less threatening as she had previous experience of it and she agreed. Whilst this may not have been totally necessary, it gave the midwife time alone with her in a situation that was familiar and not threatening.*

*Asked about the father of the child, Kara explained her mother's hostility towards him and how she met him secretly, so getting pregnant by him had caused a lot of family hurt and anger. Kara felt that she could deal with this but wanted it to remain confidential, as she felt her mother was controlling so much of her life. Helping Kara to see she had choices and a space for herself helped her feel more in control.*

Sometimes, women are afraid to tell anyone what is happening, fearing their responses or just not knowing how to manage the future.

*Gemma was a 16-year-old girl living at home with her parents who both worked full time; and a younger brother still at school. She had just started work, having decided that she did not want to go to university, although her school had encouraged that. She realised she was pregnant by a casual boyfriend at around 12 weeks. She decided not to tell anyone in the hope that it might all go away. A plump girl, she managed to hide the pregnancy to almost full term, when she went into labour alone at home. She phoned an aunt, who then called an ambulance. The baby was delivered at home and then she was taken to hospital.*

*Gemma was terrified of telling her parents and asked the midwife to be there when they arrived, summoned by the aunt. All the family were shocked and concerned. The midwife was able to reassure them about Gemma's and the baby's health and what support they might expect. Gemma was relieved to find they were not angry with her; but rather hurt that she had not told them. A close, large family they rallied round her and decided that they could manage another baby in the family.*

*Difficulties came when social services were called because of Gemma's age and the hidden pregnancy. The family resented this and saw it as a slur on their ability to "look after our own". Relationships with all the professionals were threatened and took some time to repair.*

The first contact women have with professionals may be very significant for their feelings of self and about the pregnancy. Honest reactions without assumptions and expectations make the woman feel safe, whatever her feelings about the pregnancy. Relating to the professionals as people depends on the professionals being genuine and warm, listening as much as talking and giving the woman space to talk, even in a fairly rushed situation.

*LeeAnne had been in a relationship with Ella for four years. They had decided they wanted a family two years before and had chosen a male friend as the donor. LeeAnne's family had struggled with her decision to have children but had been supportive. However, she had felt that some friends and colleagues had been judgmental about it and she had been worried about speaking to her doctor who had been her family GP from childhood. She decided not to explain the situation but invented a story that she felt would be easier. Ella was angry with her and felt that she had been betrayed. Eventually they told more friends but not the GP. This time LeeAnne felt she could be honest about the pregnancy, but she was still very reluctant to say much to the midwife, although she felt that she should not need to keep it a secret.*

*LeeAnne was very tense talking about the situation, checking with the midwife's face for any signs of disapproval or judgement. She felt she had got herself into a difficult situation and needed help to untangle it and to feel more positive about the pregnancy, rather than anxiety about the lies and uncertainty, and also the threat to the relationship.*

In all these examples of real situations and interactions, whilst the time for a midwife to engage with difficult emotional issues is short, and no one is expecting her or him to be a counsellor, there are basic counselling principles that can be used. These often get the best results in helping a client to relax and feel they can trust the midwife. "I wonder how you feel about this" may be enough of an open question to help someone feel you are interested in hearing their response.

Empathy, genuineness and non-judgmental listening all help the client to feel heard and therefore more able to express the difficult feelings that may affect a pregnancy, and so the client's willingness to comply with advice and care plans. If the client understands why certain questions are asked, they are more likely to cooperate and be less defensive. Some people will be anxious about anything that is recorded about them. Understanding and accepting the reason for the question and who will share the information will help the communication.

## TALKING ABOUT UNCERTAINTY

Early scans, possible problems and multiple pregnancies all bring changes to how the pregnancy is thought about and how the professionals need to communicate with the clients.

*Sheila and John were shocked to see two babies at their first scan. Sheila had an early scan as she had had some bleeding at 7 weeks. They came out of the scan room in shock. This was not what they had planned and the thought of managing twins was overwhelming to them both. This seemed quite unusual to the midwife until they explained to her their family history.*

*John was one of twins. The pregnancy for his mother had not gone well and his twin died in utero. John had many unresolved feelings about this and as his mother had now died there was nowhere to take his worries and anxieties. Sheila became very anxious what would happen to her: would history repeat itself why had it happened to her mother in law? There were no answers for them so they both needed to be supported during the pregnancy by listening to their anxieties and acknowledging them. One-to-one care would have offered them the support they required to manage the uncertainty during the pregnancy. Also, the support organisation Twins and Multiple Birth Association (TAMBA) have telephone support lines which can be accessed both during pregnancy and after birth.*

## ECTOPIC PREGNANCY

When no pregnancy sac can be seen in the uterus of a woman with a positive pregnancy test, then further investigations will be performed. Suspicion will point to a possible ectopic pregnancy and uncertainty creates heightened anxiety. Breaking the news about a possible ectopic pregnancy will most usually fall to those who scan in Early Pregnancy (Assessment) Units (EPU/EPAU) and do not see a pregnancy sac in the uterus. There is little preparation for them, other than the symptoms women present with, which may heighten their suspicion. It is recognised that uncertainty will increase women's anxiety.

EPUs have been set up to provide privacy, dignity, sensitivity and supportive care. These units are expected to be a dedicated service provided by healthcare professionals competent to diagnose and care for women with pain and/or bleeding in early pregnancy; to offer ultrasound and assessment of serum human chorionic gonadotrophin (hCG) levels; and be staffed by healthcare professionals with training in sensitive communication and breaking bad news (NICE Clinical Guidelines, No. 154.2012). Women who require referral should be given information about why the referral was necessary and what they might expect when they arrive at the EPU. Staff will continue to offer information and support throughout the care they provide. In helping her to understand what their diagnosis means; professionals need to use words with which the woman is familiar. Medical terms can be unfamiliar and confusing. This becomes more complicated if there are language difficulties. Asking clients what they understand about what they have been told helps to know what they have heard and ensure the information is appropriate to them. If their questions or worries are on technical issues, offering the information or directing them to someone who can provide an answer often helps.

Listening skills will help the professional to determine how to help the woman. Support through this time will be vital to the woman's experience of her care. Focusing on her emotional needs will demonstrate support and, whilst psychological support appears to be important, there are no specific details for the professionals to help them, especially when they are dealing with the distress after delivering bad news.

Women diagnosed with an ectopic pregnancy may have additional negative consequences, both physical and emotional. In addition to the emotional reactions to the loss of a pregnancy and baby, women undergo unwanted surgical intervention to end a pregnancy. If they are unwell, as can be expected if the ectopic causes physical symptoms, there will be anxiety for the woman's health. Internal bleeding from a ruptured ectopic can be very dramatic and even life-threatening. The loss of control and fear of death can be very frightening for the woman and her family.

*Staff caring for the woman can also be affected by the seriousness of the situation and value the support of Specialist Midwives to offer them, their client and her family the emotional support they need. Supporting a woman through this dissonance enables other themes of loss to emerge and the full impact of the event to be experienced. Around the time of surgery, care will be directed to saving the life of the woman, which is a scary situation for the family. Afterwards, they often concentrate on this factor, whilst the woman is grieving for her pregnancy. Kitty told the counsellor that she had been 12 weeks pregnant when, 4 weeks ago, she was admitted to A and E with pain in her shoulder and intermittent bleeding. The next thing she recalled was being rushed to theatre after being told she had an ectopic pregnancy and needed surgery. As the details emerged, tears fell from her eyes and she began to shake.*

*It appeared to the counsellor that Kitty had felt disconnected from what was happening to her but in the telling of her story, she was re-experiencing the fear she had felt about what was clearly an emergency situation. Kitty recalled her family looked very frightened and afterwards they cried and told her how lucky she was to be alive. The nursing and medical staff reflected this too and no-one had talked to her about the loss of her pregnancy. She felt this aspect had been discounted by them all and she had had no permission to grieve for the loss of her baby.*

*The counsellor offered Kitty her reflection about the disconnection and it seemed to make sense. As Kitty explored what this pregnancy had meant for her, she was also able to reflect on the frightening situation she had experienced. It also served as momentum for returning to see the medical staff to have some practical questions answered in the pursuit of psychological resolution.*

## RESEARCH ON ECTOPIC PREGNANCY

In a prospective cohort study following women with pregnancy loss at an EPU in London, Farren[18] concluded that after an ectopic pregnancy, some women did demonstrate particular symptoms of PTSD (Post Traumatic Stress Disorder). These persisted for three months after their pregnancy loss. Benute[19], in looking at the risk of suicide following ectopic pregnancy, saw depression, anxiety, stress and guilt connected to an increased risk of suicide ideation symptoms. Detecting these ongoing risks, evaluating and referring for therapy depends on the knowledge of the caregivers in the community.

At present there is little or no research on what interventions would improve psychological outcomes for women following ectopic pregnancy. A small study in Australia by Catherine Chojenta[20] looked at all types of pregnancy loss in an attempt to gather enough information about mental health issues raised by loss. Their findings indicated that women who experience loss should be targeted for the assessment of mental health problems after the loss and also during any further pregnancy. It did not offer any guidance about which strategies would be helpful.

## ECTOPIC PREGNANCY AND THE PROFESSIONAL

NICE clinical guideline No. 154. 2012. supports staff in offering appropriate emotional support and recognises that "emotional support is not the same thing as formal counselling". Emotional displays of behaviour can overwhelm staff, who feel at a loss themselves and are uncertain how to manage such situations. The value of "being with the distress" cannot be overestimated. However, the professional desire to make the situation better conflicts with allowing the distress to be expressed. It often feels safer for the professional to move on with explanations and referral to a doctor, but this can be too much information too quickly delivered to be of use. Recognising that this news has been a shock and then leaving space for the woman to ask the questions she needs answering can help to move her on to have those questions answered by the appropriate professional.

After these difficult conversations, reviewing what worked and what did not can help the professional with the conflict. A non-judgmental space to explore what emotional reactions were evoked in the professional can provide a deeper understanding of their individual responses to a stressful situation and also offer positive reinforcement. When staff recognise that counselling could be of benefit, therapy services are not always easily available. Sourcing appropriate psychological therapy, which may not be NHS funded, depends on local services. Counsellors who work in hospitals will be able to offer direction to staff. The patients' GPs may have access to counselling either at the surgery or may have local contacts.

Signposting women and their families to the professional body for counselling and psychotherapy (bacp.co.uk) may help them to find the help they need. Charities and voluntary organisations such as the Miscarriage Association and the Ectopic Trust are also sources of excellent literature and have support lines for online discussions and counselling. These sources of support can bring comfort from being with others experiencing similar emotions.

## MOLAR PREGNANCY

Molar pregnancy, also known as Gestational Trophoblastic Disease (GTD), is an extremely rare form of non-viable pregnancy. The trophoblastic cells develop in the uterus when fertilisation has been abnormal. This is still a very rare complication of pregnancy, so few women will have heard of it, let alone what the management will be. Diagnosis will take place in the EPU and the women will be shocked at the news and will need time to absorb the information that their pregnancy will not continue. The information contained in the 'breaking bad news' section of this book will help the professional to deliver the news face-to-face in a compassionate manner. It is important that there is written information to hand to support what has been said.

If surgery to remove the cells can be performed, the cells will be taken out and examined, and pregnancy tests repeated until there is a negative result. Medical treatment relies on the use of chemotherapy treatment, which does have side effects. The use of these drugs in a fertility setting can be shocking news to women and their partners. There may be a reluctance to take the drugs because of the side effects. The medication offered will take time to work and there may be no definite ending to the pregnancy for weeks. Any further pregnancy is contraindicated for quite a lengthy time. Staff can be challenged about the best way to both address the above and offer continuing support through the time it takes for the drugs to affect the cells and the pregnancy to end. The giving of factual and practical information in the form of patient support leaflets is easier for the multidisciplinary team to offer, but the support required may well extend further into managing the many complex feelings that will arise.

Whilst fears and feelings fluctuate throughout treatment, staff caring for women will need to be flexible and responsive to issues and questions as they arise. At some points, there will be almost daily contact for medical reasons. Staff will not know how a woman's emotions are changing throughout the experience unless they check.

For those who do not have access to face-to-face meetings (for example, those who live far away on remote islands), the use of phone real time calls such as Skype can help give much-needed continuing support.

If women raise questions to which the professional does not have the answer, it is generally fine to say you don't know, but always offer to find out with a timescale and make sure you do get back to them with the correct information in a timely fashion.

Coping with the emotions of women, their partners and families over the weeks during treatment demands counselling skills that can be tested during the time it takes to resolve the pregnancy. Answering questions openly and honestly and holding on to any expressed anxieties with the woman and her family will help both her and them to feel confident in their care.

In the UK there are specialist centres of care but the local team on the spot may be easier to access and so many queries will be directed their way. Whilst GTD is curable and there will be a full recovery, women will be confronting the loss of the pregnancy; facing taking cytotoxic drugs, with the resulting side effects; and a wait to even try to get pregnant again. There will be a heightened anxiety when that pregnancy happens, and ongoing psychological care must be based on awareness of the complex emotions women and their families will suffer.

## RESEARCH ON MOLAR PREGNANCY: PSYCHOLOGICAL SEQUELAE

As this is a rare condition, the studies published contain small samples. Valentina Di Mattei et al[21] questioned 37 patients in Milan focusing on "perceived fertility, depression and anxiety". Whilst there were many variables in terms of their research and they acknowledge the limitations, they concluded their findings highlighted the need for including a psychological component to the clinical management.

The works of Rodney W Peterson[22] and Lari Wenzel[23] both recognised the psychological impact of a GTD and pointed to a need for greater support for these women, which Peterson concluded could be offered by a multi-disciplinary team. In a systematic review into Health Related Quality of Life (HRQOL) Jane Ireson *et al*[24] concluded that, whilst most research has been concerned with physical sequelae, more comprehensive research concerning HRQOL would help to establish what supportive care and care pathways would best support both women and their partners during active treatment and monitoring, and to determine what their needs are for the longer-term consequences of both the disease and their ongoing fertility.

The RCOG publishes patient information on molar pregnancy but does not offer any contacts for psychological support. Molarpregnancy.co.uk is a community website with professional counsellors available who can offer the psychological help when staff feel clients need more skilled support

## LONGER TERM EFFECTS OF EARLY LOSS

There is some evidence that suffering a loss may have an effect on the mother's attachment to future children. Heller and Zeanah[25] in the Infant Mental Health Journal looked at mothers who had delivered a child within 19 months of a perinatal loss and found that 45% had some disorganised attachments to the new baby. There is insufficient research in this area, and it is important not to generalise from the small samples available.

The effect on the father may also be underestimated as he, too, has lost a child and is experiencing a change to his future, as well as wanting to support his partner. Men will often be reluctant to talk about it and may continue to work without telling colleagues. This can sometimes leave a painful space with feelings of loss and readjustment, as well as some fear for future pregnancies.

Fathers and same-sex partners sometimes talk about feeling they have "lost" the woman after an early pregnancy loss. They are not sure how to reach her and to talk about what has happened. They may also be anxious about initiating sex, although that may make them feel closer. The mother may want this or may feel she needs space or does not want to risk another pregnancy. Encouragement to talk about this may stop them both feeling that the other is not understanding their needs.

Sometimes the whole family may be affected, as potential grandparents have also lost the shared future and may find it hard at first to adjust to the loss. Siblings, too, may feel the loss if they knew a baby was on the way. Encouraging people to talk about it and to recognise that they are not to blame may help them to look forward. Many women try to work out what they may have done wrong, if they exercised too much or too little, had a drink, went out with friends or worked late. These are all ways of trying to explain to oneself what may be inexplicable, but they are all self-blaming and unhelpful. It can be helpful for women to understand there may not be a clear explanation and they may have to live with not knowing but not blaming.

Women may also need help in explaining the situation to their other children. Child Bereavement UK has helpful advice and leaflets around children experiencing loss. Other countries have similar organisations with details online. Corbett, Owen and Kruger[26] found that women and their partners had better psychological outcomes in terms of guilt and self-blame if they had a clear explanation of what had happened to them and the opportunity to discuss options. It was particularly helpful when health professionals could explain that there may have been nothing they could have done and that they were not to blame.

Grieving parents may need time to come to terms with what has happened and staff need to be sensitive to those who do not want to talk at that time but giving some literature or a number to call if they want to in the future, may be enough. They may not want to explore the feelings before a future pregnancy or some other life event. Validating the experience is the most valuable communication.

> *Sally came back to see the counsellor she had seen after her pregnancy loss 3 years ago. She was finally pregnant again but instead of feeling excited, she was crying and returning to thoughts about the baby she had lost. This was unnerving for her as she was not usually given to talking about feelings or displaying her emotions. She did not understand her reactions. Her family would be delighted for her, but she was fearful of hearing their positivity. Sally needed the acknowledgement that this was a normal reaction and support offering her space and time to grieve and let go of what might have been.*

Women in this position feel frightened to invest again in the hope of the future, which can affect the next pregnancy, when they can experience a sense of loss all over again. This anxiety does not go away after a successful pregnancy and birth, so often care will have to be tailored to individual needs in further pregnancies too.

Fear during a subsequent pregnancy is a natural response. When the psyche tries to negotiate living with bad things that have happened, it begins to fear they will happen again. With positive affirmation of the reality of the fears and anxieties and support, Sally started to allow herself to look forward again. This may be a time when an appointments and scans not usually scheduled in a pregnancy can be very useful. When the first few months have been successfully negotiated, the baby starts to move and, in the woman's mind, to develop their own personality, then this task can be undertaken.

Sally recognised this baby as "moving very differently" and so it changed in her mind to the new baby. The term "rainbow baby" is often used now to describe a successful pregnancy after a miscarriage.

In-patient miscarriages and terminations may be nursed on a ward where the staff may have little time to deal with the emotional effects of the event. Nurses in England may be expected to care for women on medical/surgical wards and may not have any training or support with managing all the emotional needs of the family.

In a study by Chan[27] et al in the Journal of Advanced Nursing, nurses reported feeling that they were dealing with the women's medical and emotional needs and also having to deal with their own responses to the situation. A qualitative study by Murphy and Merrell[28] identified the differences between how nurses would like to practise in the area of early pregnancy loss and the reality of working on a ward. They felt that they understood the women's needs but were frustrated at not being able to meet them, because of time constraints, financial pressures, and/or lack of support and training.

A study by Roehrs in the USA[29] looked at the needs of nurses dealing with perinatal loss. One of the most significant areas was their concern about the lack of training and ongoing support. They felt they lacked expertise in this area and that, whilst they wanted to be calm and open and answer questions clearly, they were concerned about saying or doing the wrong thing and this compromised their ability to give individualised care at the level they thought was necessary. Many midwives may only deal with the after-effects of miscarriage when they see a woman for a subsequent pregnancy. This may be the first time that the woman has talked about her loss, perhaps to anyone, but almost certainly to a professional carer. Giving genuine attention to her fears and feelings may help her to express them.

There are Early Pregnancy Units in around 200 NHS hospitals which do give staff the opportunity to focus more on emotional needs and support, as well as developing expertise in the area.

## FINDING INFORMATION AND SUPPORT

It has become much easier, with the development of the internet, to find information and support online. It may not always be easy to judge the accuracy of the information but there are reliable sites that can help at all stages of pregnancy. These are outlined in a future chapter. For those considering a termination, there is guidance as to where to go and what to expect but there are also sites that are anti-abortion and may frighten or mislead women at a vulnerable time. There are online - and some telephone - groups where women can find support from others who have shared the experience at all stages of pregnancy. Many women find it immensely helpful to be able to read about other people's experiences and advice, or to have anonymous contact with others.

Healthcare professionals will find practical information from their professional bodies' websites but help in coping with both the clients' emotional needs and their own needs may not be so readily available. These are detailed at the end of the book. There are groups and advice centres available throughout the country where women can meet others for support and information and sometimes for friendship. These may not be widespread, particularly in rural areas, which makes the internet very valuable. Many GP surgeries and antenatal clinics will have information about local services.

# 3: The Second Trimester: 12 to 24 weeks

*Ultrasound scans; informed choice; declining screening; false positives/negatives; diagnostic testing; giving results by phone; making decisions; continuing with a pregnancy; mid-trimester spontaneous miscarriage; psychological outcomes; the 20-week scan; issues around loss at 20-24 weeks; professional reactions to loss at 20-24 weeks; follow-on care.*

The medical epidemiology of mid-trimester loss has been described by Regan and Rai[1]. They estimate that miscarriage after a foetal heart has been seen in the first trimester and after the 12th week affects 1-2% of all pregnancies. The ending of a pregnancy between 12 and 24 weeks may be spontaneous, induced after a diagnosis of abnormality or induced due to death in utero. It is most definitely not expected.

> *I couldn't wait to let people know that we were pregnant and we were very excited to see our little babe. Nothing prepared me for the news that was given to me by the sonographer. I could tell from the silence that something was not right, but nothing can prepare you for this news. She said, "I am sorry, but your baby is not the right size for your dates and I am unable to find a heartbeat". She then asked a colleague to come and scan me and he confirmed her findings. "What does not seeing the heartbeat mean?", I asked them. Only then did she tell me it meant the baby had died.*

> *I was so shocked and did not really understand that information. I was unable to speak. I am so glad my partner was with me because he was able to ask the questions I could not even frame in my mind.*

The professional could have helped at the beginning of the conversation by preparing the way, adding the information that no heartbeat probably did mean the baby had died and that it was important to have this checked out by another sonographer. This allows some time for the woman to consider the meaning of these words and prepare herself or her partner to ask questions at the time. This may be a first experience of loss and any first-time experience involves uncertainty about the feelings. There are no 'right' or 'wrong' feelings: just the ones that are there. Allowing them to be expressed helps to normalise them. It may be scary, confusing, frightening and difficult to talk about.

The professional holding on through this confusion can do much to help just by listening and sticking with the feelings as they are expressed. There are often complex issues that are raised by the situation and knowing it is ok to express them helps to clarify for the individual what to prioritise. This is not a problem-solving exercise for the professional but offering empathy and respect goes a long way.

> *Through her tears, Pam explained that she did not want to lose her baby. She said she had not wanted to be pregnant at first and in fact, had denied it. By then, it was too late to have a termination. Contact with the midwife/GP had not uncovered this ambivalence, which she had kept hidden from the professionals. Now it was all flowing out as she opened up with a very junior member of the medical team, whilst she was being advised about what would happen next, now it had been confirmed the pregnancy had ended. Many thoughts were going through her head, including the question had she brought this about through her negative reaction to her pregnancy? The doctor was reassuring but this did not help her.*

> *Talking this situation through with the nurse later, the subject of ambivalent reactions to pregnancy arose. Pam said she had started her pregnancy unexpectedly and was very uncertain about how she would manage as a single mother. Even whilst she was denying the pregnancy, she was also thinking about how changed her future would be. As she passed the 12 weeks mark, she began to see a way that could work for her. Having done all this work, only to find out the pregnancy was not viable, raised her concern that somehow, she had bought this about herself. This kind of magical thinking is not unusual and comes from an inner belief that one's own thoughts, wishes or desires can influence the external world. The thought processes that created the belief may be very strong. If this is the way Pam addresses other problems in her life, changing her thought processes can only come about if she realises the steps that led her into this thought pattern are not helping her and she chooses to make changes.*

There are even more complex challenges if there have been fertility problems and getting pregnant has involved sometimes complicated treatments. Women emerging from this experience become psychologically acclimatized to loss through repeated cycles that did not end in a pregnancy. Worry and anxiety are a part of the pregnancy experience but in these situations the emotions may well be heightened. Failure of a pregnancy leads to a sense of self-criticism, loss of belief that the body can support a pregnancy and fear about a changed future. Anticipating there will be repeated loss, women may react unexpectedly, especially at the 12-week scan.

When there has been a previous pregnancy loss, there will also be fear of repeated loss and anxiety. Managing these complex emotional reactions demands specialist input. Sonographers are highly skilled in their speciality and will need to have some awareness of coping with different and often complex emotions. Background knowledge about why such emotions as denial and fear are present - that they are normal reactions to differing situations - may help to support their work.

*Gemma had been attending a fertility clinic for five years, during which time she had undergone many investigations, leading to three IVF attempts. Two of these had failed and now this last cycle had resulted in a pregnancy. Her partner Jack had already said he could not go through any further treatment so there was extreme pressure on this pregnancy to be successful. She had had scans at six and eight weeks, which confirmed the pregnancy.*

*The eight-week scan at the fertility clinic was set up because Gemma was very anxious and had called the clinic several times with her worries. By the time she attended for her 12-week scan, she felt quite confident that all would be well. The scan went well, and she agreed to be screened as per the protocol, without really considering the implications. When she was told the result that she had a high ratio for the baby having Edwards Syndrome, she was devastated.*

*She returned to the fertility counsellor she had seen during her time at the clinic, who had helped her with mobilising coping strategies. The shock she was experiencing was causing her to panic and this disrupted her thinking. Sitting with her distress allowed her to express all the thoughts that were teeming through her head. When the outpouring of all these thoughts and emotions ended, she was quiet and looked exhausted. The counsellor could then engage with her. Over the next sessions Gemma worked through her options, decided with her partner to go for diagnosis with amniocentesis and made plans for the potential outcomes.*

*Here the counsellor was able to hold her anxieties so that she could then consider clearly how she could work through the next steps. She did not give Gemma a way through but by listening and validated her anxieties, Gemma could then work out her own way through these dilemmas.*

In all the above scenarios, 'miscarriage' is the more common term used by all professional teams, rather than the older, more technical but loaded term of 'abortion'; but this term can implicitly suggest that *the woman* did something wrong (i.e. I miscarried) and so carries a negative meaning and introduces the emotion of guilt.

"I lost my baby" can sound dramatic to those who have not lived through each hour and week of the pregnancy, but the mental picture of the baby is much more real when seen on scan at early gestations. Women often express a sense of "safety" after the scan. After all, they can see arms, legs, a beating heart, the head and body; so now they can really visualise their developing baby. The baby becomes more real in the parents' eyes and now takes on a kind of personhood. The shock of loss at this stage can be profound and deep. Unexpected emotions may surface which the professionals dealing with the miscarriage may find difficult. At the time of the scan, they are not able to fully understand all the individual factors that go towards the attachment to this pregnancy.

Disbelief at the news is commonly accompanied by the question, "Are you sure?" and this can be felt as a challenge to the professional. Showing the scan of the baby, explaining where the heartbeat should be seen and asking another professional to confirm there is no heartbeat may help to ensure clarity of information and helps give validity for the professional. The shock may prevent other emotions flooding in straight away. As the reality of the news sinks in, so does the realisation that the loss of the pregnancy also means the future has been taken away and all the dreams and hopes are gone. The emotions experienced at this time are individual and unique, but they are also common to all those who mourn.

## ULTRASOUND SCANS

After the scan between 11 and 13 weeks, which may be the first scan in the pregnancy, the next set of challenges in managing the pregnancy commences.

The use of scans in early pregnancy does mean that women have to confront loss in unfamiliar, almost always public places. This will be a distressing event and can lead to very strong reactions. All pregnant women in the UK and many other countries are offered screening and there is a sense that screening is 'routine', as reflected in Benzie[2]. Many women view it more as an opportunity to see the baby rather than as a part of the screening process.

For the professional, one part of the purpose of the scan at this time is to date the pregnancy and check for nuchal translucency, which along with blood tests, forms the national screening programme for mother and baby, as set out by the Department of Health UK National Screening Committee Guidelines.

Explaining the screening and choices to be made is a difficult task for staff who are unfamiliar with non-directive practice. The conversations undertaken at this time about the process and the implications of the tests may not be fully understood, as they are often overshadowed by the excitement of the scan. Women are given written information about all the screening procedures and invited to ask questions.

Those who have communication problems for whatever reasons are encouraged to make decisions, but they may not be able to read or understand the literature they are given. They may be embarrassed or unwilling to talk with the professionals about their lack of comprehension; and it is not appropriate to have a family member translate and interpret for them, because it cannot then be assumed that the information given is correct and that the woman is making her own choice. Using professional interpreters helps to ensure women have the opportunity to ask questions and that the decisions they are making are their own.

The concept of screening can be difficult to fully understand and the implications of these tests and potential decisions may pose real ethical and moral dilemmas for the women, their partners and the staff caring for them. The tests and resulting decisions present challenges for the clinician.

Ledward[3] recognises that in order for women to have autonomy in their decision-making, midwives need support to enable them to be non-judgemental and objective when giving information about the programme. In other words, a counselling approach will offer women the chance to make their own decisions. Medical science is continually refining tests that can give detailed information about the structural and genetic status of the baby. This in turn introduces pregnant women to the difficult concept of screening, and to the risks and decisions to be made. There can also be couple differences; and the influences of family culture and religion all play their part.

# INFORMED CHOICE

In a review of both qualitative and quantitative research on the factors that influence parents in the take up of testing for Down's Syndrome, Skirton and Barr[4] identified that sometimes, healthcare professionals were not fully prepared and competent to offer all the information about the implications of screening. This alone may diminish the opportunity for open discussion about informed choice. For example, women may ask questions about Down's Syndrome to which the professionals may not have answers. When women want to know more, it is highly appropriate to refer to someone with a greater depth of knowledge, who can authoritatively provide answers. Literature on screening and the further information available is also online and could be offered so that the decision to have the test or not is made only when the woman feels she has had time to digest the information and equipped to make her own informed decision.

Spreading the news of a pregnancy is often initiated after the scan at 12 weeks and posted on social media. The secret weeks are now over, and this is the starting point for telling family, friends, work colleagues and the wider world of social networking about the baby. Messages are received and more information is shared, such as the due date. Suddenly, the pregnancy is made very public.

Inevitably, the loss of a pregnancy after this time then becomes very public. Women are often surprised to learn from their family and friends that others have suffered the same fate, which demonstrates that women prefer to keep their fertility journey private and not share the experiences they do not feel good about. Whilst sometimes this can increase anxiety about the frequency of pregnancy loss within the community, hearing about it can help to normalise their situation and enable them to learn how others have dealt with their own loss. Everyone selects consciously or unconsciously who they trust to give them information. For many, this is the professionals. Others feel that people who have had similar experiences are more able to understand, empathise and support them, and so will turn to the internet or support groups.

> *After Rosie miscarried one of the things that was difficult for her was informing the friends she had told about the pregnancy on social media. When she did, she was surprised to hear back from friends who had also suffered pregnancy loss but had never shared this information with her before. Rosie found talking about these feelings with her friends helped her to see her feelings were not abnormal but were shared by many others.*

Using social media at this time can help to confirm the normality of feelings but there are no filters, so encouraging access may lead to more confusion and distress if the posts received refer to individual circumstances that differ greatly from the experience of the woman. Also, once the information is public, it cannot be retracted, and the woman may feel exposed without support.

There are many reasons women choose not to talk about their pregnancy loss. They may have chosen to terminate the pregnancy for social or medical reasons, or miscarried spontaneously before telling anyone about the pregnancy. Women reveal that sometimes it is guilt which keeps them from sharing with others. Guilt is often experienced around loss. Women feel they have done something wrong - maybe had a glass of wine, ate some cheese or behaved in a way that had put their pregnancy at risk.

Professionals often rush to reassure women this is not the case but an approach which also includes talking about normal feelings after loss is valuable to their ongoing emotional recovery. Guilt is a normal part of grief. Acknowledging this can allow the woman to let go of the anxiety associated with the experiencing the guilt.

## ANTENATAL DIAGNOSTIC PROCEDURES

The UK National Screening Committee guidelines[5] state the information discussed with parents should include:

- The rationale for offering screening

- Information that the screening tests are optional

- Types of screening offered

- False positive and false negative rates associated with the tests

- Diagnostic tests available if screening test results indicate a high risk

- Limitations of the screening tests

- The way in which the results are conveyed to the parents

- Options available if the foetus is diagnosed with a genetic condition, including discussing termination

All this information can be overwhelming, both for the giver and the receiver, and can lead to complex discussions. Although checklists can be used to ensure all the information has been given, there is little emphasis on checking the understanding of those who do not like to ask questions. All this can also be uncomfortable for the professionals, who are unprepared for such detailed and time-consuming discussions in their busy daily routines.

Communicating information accurately and honestly, in a genuine and empathetic way, with time allowed for questions, is vital to encourage good relations. Communication between doctors, nurses and all healthcare staff can be crucial to meeting patients' expectations. The team seen to be working together with sensitivity and a clear understanding of individual responsibilities will offer care that leads to greater patient satisfaction.

Women have differing influences on their decision-making processes that are unknown to the clinician. Each woman is unique, with her own set of personal, social, ethical, religious and moral values. Providing the information they require to help them make a decision demands recognition of varying levels of knowledge and skill in conveying information. Giving all this information to women and their families and checking their understanding demands great communication skills. Add to this the complication of language differences and the task becomes even more complex.

> *Serena was taking the booking history for Becca. When she began to talk about the screening tests, Becca asked for more detailed information about what women decide to do. Next, Becca asked Serena what she would do. Suddenly, the barrier of the professional and the personal had been breached. It can be very easy to offer a personal response but this avoids making an individual decision. Instead of either sharing or declining to give that information, Serena led the conversation further by asking, "I am wondering if making this decision is difficult for you? Can you tell me why?". Becca talked about what friends and family had been telling her and appeared to place little value on her own voice. It was clear to Serena that if she had offered her opinion it may have led Becca into making a decision that was not her own. In encouraging Becca to explore her own thoughts about this subject, Serena was helping her to make her own decisions and not to be led by the voices of others.*

## DECLINING SCREENING

There will be women who read the screening information and take the decision not to be tested. Some women would not contemplate ending a pregnancy for any reason. Amongst their reasons will be their preference not to know about any problems with their baby and a certainty that they would not end the pregnancy anyway. This decision will probably not have been arrived at without a great deal of thought and discussion and may have been questioned already by worried family members.

In the NHS public health functions agreement 2017-18 Service Specification no. 15 NHS Infectious Diseases in Pregnancy Screening Programme (IDPS), the following standard concerning screening is explained. At the first offer of screening the healthcare professional should:

> *"discuss her decision to decline and ensure that she is fully apprised of the benefits of screening for IDPS for her and their baby, re-offer the screening test and, if accepted, arrange testing and follow up of the result. If the woman declines the second formal re-offer of screening, the local multidisciplinary team will be responsible for further management. In line with local clinical protocols the onus of the reoffer is to facilitate an informed choice and not to coerce women to accept screening."*

Whilst most women do accept screening at some point in their pregnancy, the challenge some healthcare professionals and families face, is to accept the decision of those who continue to decline the offer and try to understand their reasons.

> *After Omar was born, he was diagnosed with Down's Syndrome and sadly he did have an associated heart problem. The paediatric team leading his care were concerned that his mother had declined screening and asked for an investigation into how this had happened. The midwife who booked his mother was seen to find out how she had handled and recorded the situation.*

> *The midwife came to see the counsellor in tears. She did recall the woman and had taken advice and support from the Specialist Midwife. All the guidelines were followed and the recording of the discussions that had taken place was appropriate. Even so, she wondered if she could have done more. The discussion continued around what constitutes informed consent and what is coercion. She also found it difficult to accept the information she had given had not brought about change in the mother's decision. In this situation, it can be difficult to stand with the woman and accept her reasons.*

# FALSE POSITIVES AND FALSE NEGATIVES

Because screening does not reveal a positive or negative result, women will continue with pregnancies believing all is well, since their risk of having an affected baby is low, only to be shocked when later on, they discover a problem at birth.

*After his wife had given birth to a son with Down's Syndrome, Danny, the father, became very angry, demanding of the screening coordinator why we had not detected this in the antenatal period. She advised them that the results of the blood test had given a risk over 1/300. The cut-off in England for further investigative tests is 1/150. This meant no further tests would have been recommended. The professionals involved are trained to help them to fully understand what this risk means but families often do not understand it. At this time, the professionals will be helping women, their partners and families to come to terms with the outcome. Anger and resentment are common reactions to hearing the diagnosis, which also disturbs the relationship with the baby. Danny was feeling very distressed and could see the tough choices ahead for the family. Understandably, he had many practical questions and directing him to the support he required was fundamental to his need to cope with this experience.*

*The professionals involved were experiencing difficult emotions, too: feeling anxious and challenged by his anger and wanting to defend what they felt as an attack with the available facts. Silences can feel very uncomfortable in these situations, so the temptation is to fill the silence with information. It became clear that the information given to the couple before the tests failed to help them to understand that screening is not an exact science. What level of checking of their understanding was undertaken before the test?*

*Those in pain with grief want to apportion blame and the focus in this case was the screening tests because it appeared the parents expected any abnormality to be picked up. Danny said that if they had known early in the pregnancy, they would been equipped to make the decision whether or not to continue.*

*These initial reactions were not only disturbing the first few weeks of bonding with this baby but could impact on the child's future, because the whole family dynamics had been changed forever. Both mother and father were exhibiting very normal symptoms of grief and loss. This baby was not what they were expecting and as the shock subsided, the tasks of mourning began. Support for this couple needed to be focused on recognising their loss with a non-judgemental and empathetic approach. Angry reactions can be uncomfortable to hear but need space for expression by those learning to live with this devastating situation.*

*The staff trying to help the couple understand how this could have happened became defensive when faced with anger and disappointment. Their focus was to explain the implications of the tests in early pregnancy and the concept of screening. This may have felt more comfortable for the staff but only increased his anger and alienation.*

*Danny did not feel at all heard. On reflection, the staff could have allowed Danny to have the voice he needed, to consider what was really going on and allow him to be angry about the changed circumstances for himself and his family. Knowledge about how both women and men exhibit normal reactions grief and loss could have helped them in the interaction with the parents, enabling them to understand Danny's anger and recognised how deeply this had changed his circumstances.*

Screening does not give a simple yes or no answer. Women receive a risk factor for which no further tests will be needed but some (approximately 5%) will be given a result that leads to decisions about diagnostic testing. Considerations around decision-making will be explored in a further chapter.

## DIAGNOSTIC TESTING

When screening leads to further tests and a diagnosis is confirmed, women and their partners will be faced with very tough decisions. The continuing development of tests and diagnostic procedures lead parents towards finding out even more information about their baby. Whilst this seems to offer them more choices as individuals, it also leads to ethical, moral and cultural issues that can challenge them. This is unknown territory for anyone not used to dealing with these dilemmas. Their culture and their belief system may not support them in their individual deliberations and decisions. In these life-changing situations, they may have nowhere and no-one to turn to and so feel very alone. If the culture and faith systems differ within the couple, this can lead to an even greater sense of being alone. The health professionals can answer questions and offer accurate information. Organisations are able to offer support but ultimately, it is their decision about which course to follow. In order to support women, couples and their families at this time professionals can use listening skills and reflection.

*Raiza and Gerry were not expecting the call from the midwife now advising them that the results of the screening showed their baby may have an anomaly. The words used can be frightening and the phone call was really difficult for Raiza. When she and Gerry came in to discuss these results further with the obstetrician, they had clearly done their homework and had very relevant questions. Understanding their options, they went away to consider their decision.*

*They returned to see a counsellor they had previously worked with to help them with their dilemma. This pregnancy had been a long time in coming and had been assisted by donor sperm. Feelings of guilt on both sides were expressed. Raiza was blaming herself, Gerry and her choice of donor. The couple went back to how and why they had made the decision to have a child together in an attempt to settle their feelings.*

*They were able with the counsellor to explore their feelings around the loss of a perfect child. This loss was felt profoundly by Gerry, as she had a cousin with Downs Syndrome who had not survived because of severe heart problems. Her experiences with genetic abnormalities was very much colouring the way they were both thinking about their future. Women and their partners do not always discuss their attitudes to genetic problems before they are faced with them. They may not even be aware of their partners background enough to know how they are going to react in this situation. This couple had thought that, after the 12-week scan, they were safe to tell others about their pregnancy. Now, issues of disclosure were also causing them worry. They felt safe talking to the counsellor and expressing individual thought processes. They said it really helped each of them to air their feelings, listen to and understand each other, to consider as much as they could, and both move on to make the decision that would change their lives. Supporting them through this minefield demanded careful interactions.*

Whichever decision is made, the loss of the perfect baby has already happened, and this leads to what can be a complicated grieving process that needs acknowledgment by the professionals. The consequences of making a decision will stay with them forever.

Expertise for managing these discussions demands more advanced counselling techniques. Whilst Foetal Medicine Units will have access to trained genetic counsellors who can provide clients with the information they need, it is in the counselling space that they can explore their feelings. It is there they can come to their decision, sometimes called "the least-worst decision".

NHS information does recognise this and, in its leaflet 'If antenatal screening tests find something' advises women to get as much information as they can and to contact the support organisation Antenatal Results and Choices (ARC). This charity was started to help women in these difficult situations. Their literature is freely available in Antenatal Clinics and links to their website in literature given out to all pregnant women in England. They have support lines and open chats lines for those who are able to work with phone conversations and internet contact.

This can help but can also lead to pressure to go along with others' decisions - what would you do in our place? A question to which the answer may not be ultimately helpful. This is a decision to be made by individuals taking into account their very unique circumstances and histories. Other information can be sought and is readily available on the websites focusing on pregnancy. Some women are prepared for all the events and may have already considered their views on tests, and the questions they would ask. This can help them to come to further appointments with professionals having already decided the action they want to take.

When language differences hamper the giving of information, it is always wise to use trained interpreters in every meeting with professionals. Gaining confidence in openly airing feelings can be difficult in cultures where men make the decisions for their women. If possible, having time to talk with the woman alone may help her to understand what is happening and provide a space to voice her thoughts and feelings about her situation. Here, it may be helpful to have some practical information that can be taken to faith leaders for further discussion concerning the action to be taken. It is always very helpful to offer written practical information to take away with information on helpful websites.

*Jenny was attending for her scan and blood test. She accepted the scan but declined the blood test. During the discussion with the midwife it became apparent that her decision was more to do with the actual taking of the blood, which she found intensely difficult. Hearing this and understanding her anxiety allowed the midwife to support Jenny through the blood test and so complete the screening process. For the professionals, understanding that fear often brings angry defensive reactions and addressing the fears can help.*

## GIVING RESULTS OVER THE PHONE

In England women receive the results of the blood screening tests in the post if the results are normal but screening midwives are tasked with contacting women when a high-risk result needs to be given. Contact is usually made by phone and unsurprisingly, this is a very difficult conversation which demands skills of the information giver and is complicated by the remoteness of the person receiving the news. This complicates the communication and has an enormous impact on how the results information is received.

Consideration is necessary before the phone call of the information that must be conveyed; how to check that the person who will receive the call is in a place where she can give the news all her attention; and how to deliver it in a clear manner and what support she may have immediately. Privacy and time to digest the information may not be possible during the working day. The giver of the information should also be able to answer further technical questions. Giving time to allow for questions about what happens next and the available sources of further information on the particular circumstance helps the woman to be a little more in control of the direction of the conversation.

Attitude and communication skills have an enormous impact on how the messages are received. The information giver will not know the individual's circumstances or background. This further complicates the phone conversation. Where there will be known language difficulties, it is always advisable to have a face-to-face conversation with an interpreter present. Hospitals have official translation services which can be booked to coincide with appointments. NHS 111 offers a confidential interpreting service. More information is given in the Resources section. Some local groups offer interpreting services and some charities offer a phone service. It is difficult to check how professional they are and in some local areas it may mean using someone they know from the local community.

The professional interpreter may come from the same country as the pregnant woman but may also be from a different group, class or tribe; making trust, impartiality and confidentiality a potential problem for the client. In any interpreting situation, the client may not feel able to object and it demands skill on the part of the professional to pick up this discrepancy to enable open discussion.

# MAKING DECISIONS

Little information is available on how women evaluate the information they read on social media about pregnancy and how it affects their decision-making. The potential impact of this may require consideration and discussion with the clinicians to ensure clients have a balance of information to assist them in making their decision. Some may want further face-to-face discussion and information to help them. Women make different decisions about having further tests which will offer a diagnosis and should therefore have access to skilled help in negotiating through this time.

> *Suzy was the midwife giving the information on options to Fiona and Steve. They were struggling to decide whether they should have the diagnostic test.*
>
> *Fiona knew it carried with it a risk of miscarriage and this pregnancy had been established with assisted conception. Were they prepared to put the pregnancy in jeopardy? If their baby did have Down's Syndrome, would they terminate the pregnancy? Ethical and moral decisions are very personal, and Suzy was finding it a challenge to guide them through this without offering her own personal opinion. Helping Suzy to understand that her role as a professional was to support them whatever their decision helped her to release her personal issues. We discussed the challenge for her and the conflict she felt. Then, Suzy focused on Fiona and Steve and the need for them to make their own decision. By exploring all the options open to them without making any judgements, she could help them to decide on the next steps for them.*

In these situations, the professional is often asked, "What would you do in my place?" Answering this is never easy. Offering a personal view at this point will not help the client/s and may alienate them if the answer is not in sympathy with the client's feelings. Stating that the decision has to be theirs but that all staff will support them whatever they decide allows for a difference in opinion but offers continuing support. Also, it does not leave them alone to manage their decision.

# CONTINUING A PREGNANCY WITH A KNOWN ABNORMALITY

If the decision is to continue with the pregnancy, there are several psychological tasks to negotiate including:

- Making sense of this situation
- Facing loss of perfect baby
- Making a new relationship with this baby
- Preparing for impending loss
- Sharing with significant others
- Finding support

Counselling offers a space to work through these tasks alongside the professionals who continue to give physical care and support with appropriate contact with other members of the healthcare team as may be required after the birth of the baby.

*Meg was referred to the counsellor after one of her appointments with the obstetrician where she had expressed anxiety about managing her labour and the immediate separation from her baby. During the first session, she voiced her feelings about her baby's heart defects, which meant he would not have a chance to live if he did not receive specialist surgery very soon after birth. She had been offered a termination at the time of diagnosis as the surgery he needed may not increase his chances for survival and if he did live, he could be severely handicapped.*

*Meg spoke as if she were in a dream, which gave the counsellor insight into how she was coping with this tragic situation. Even though she had heard all that she had been told about the problems with her baby, she had not allowed herself to grieve. She was quite unsure what to grieve about, as her baby was moving and growing well. Talking about labour and birth seemed to ground her in reality. She was prepared for labour at the end of pregnancy but recognised this would be a very different labour to the one she had wanted; not for any physical reasons but because she would be meeting and saying goodbye to her baby at the same time. If he survived labour, he would be taken away immediately and she would be unable to accompany him.*

*Making her plan for how she wanted to greet and say goodbye gave Meg back a sense of control and planning her labour felt normal. In the subsequent sessions, whilst thinking through her plans, Meg seemed less in a dream and began to speak fondly about her boy. She said she felt more in touch with him and was able to be more positive about his chances for survival. Further sessions worked through such issues as:*

- *Preparing for labour and birth; and preparing the staff*
- *Neonatal care: Intensive care/transfer for treatment*
- *Getting to know the baby*
- *Being apart*
- *Finding relevant groups and getting support*

The experience of loss will sometimes evoke again very personal feelings that have been buried. Recognising this can be surprising but with counselling support it can lead to some resolution of both the past and present loss.

*After she had a miscarriage, Heidi was distressed to receive questions from social media contacts about how her pregnancy was progressing. She was feeling very low and not up to updating her status on social media. She was also avoiding contact with friends. When we talked about her feelings, they seemed to be the feelings she had as a child when her parents had separated and she felt she was to blame.*

*Heidi had no support at that time and no opportunity to talk to anyone throughout what was a very tough time for her. As there was no opportunity to work through the psychological implications at that time, when she later came up against the loss of her baby, it was likely that she would relive the same feelings.*

*Hiding away with her pain seemed to her to be a protection. That is what she had done last time; but it did not get her support to deal with her feelings about the situation.*

Initially making the links and recognising the pain helped Heidi to see what she needed to do. Explaining to women that their present feelings may evoke feelings from the past can help them to understand and manage their situation.

## MID-TRIMESTER SPONTANEOUS MISCARRIAGE

Not all miscarriages in the mid trimester have a defined cause. When there is no definite reason for the loss, "What did I do?" is a frequent question from clients which leaves the professional feeling at a loss. This can be difficult for the professional, stirring uncomfortable feelings of uselessness. In this situation, the professional may want to offer false reassurance or a solution to help clients feel better. It may be of more benefit to stay with the distress, reflecting back that this is a normal reaction in these circumstances.

Women do blame themselves for their loss and in the absence of a medical reason, they will employ blame to help explain the loss. It is useful to remind ourselves that this is a normal psychological response. Usually, it does not last for long but if this does not change over time, then consideration should be given to a referral for further psychological support. Only when there is an understanding of where this comes from can moving on with the grieving process begin.

## PSYCHOLOGICAL OUTCOMES FOLLOWING TERMINATION FOR ABNORMALITY

Small studies report some adverse psychological outcomes for women. V. Davies[6] and Kersting[7] noted significant risks for both intense and maladaptive grief reactions Nazarre[8] and PTSD for women long after the event. See more about PTSD in the specific section.

As yet, no studies have been done to ascertain the differences in psychological reactions and outcomes between surgical termination and medical termination offered in the first trimester. In the second trimester, medical termination is recommended by RCOG and offered to women in the NHS. Outside the NHS in England, some clinics are offering a choice between medical and surgical termination up to 24 weeks (BPAS information).

A study looking at the difference between couples coping and reactions White-Van Mourik[9] concluded that one of the factors giving disharmony after a loss is a lack of synchronicity within the relationship, pointing to poor communication between the couple. Difficulties in coming to terms with the loss appeared to include several other factors including "parental immaturity, inability to communicate needs, a deep-rooted lack of self-esteem, lack of supporting relationships and, for those who were suffering secondary infertility".

These were small samples and may not accurately reflect the wider community, but they do give some insight into the issues presented by this complication and can help those who will be supporting their patients through the experience.

# THE 20-WEEK SCAN

Ultrasound scans have become an integral part of the pregnancy experience in many countries. They are at the same time seen as being very reassuring and anxiety provoking. A Swedish review by M Ekelin[10] of mother's and father's views on scanning in the second trimester concluded they are important milestones in the journey towards becoming parents. Scans offer direct access to their developing baby, with real time confirmation of the life inside the womb, making them a very attractive intervention. However, women using social media report being anxious about this scan. Sometimes, this can be explained by previous experience of receiving bad news at a scan; or hearing stories of others who had poor experiences. Social media does tend to offer very personal information, both good and bad experiences, which will be received differently by each woman.

The person performing the scan may well be unaware of any history that may make the woman anxious. Asking questions about how the woman is feeling about the scan and if there are there any specific concerns can reveal important. Further, knowing the history can help the clinician to offer information about the findings in a relevant and appropriate manner. In a systematic review of women's views on pregnancy ultrasound, by Garcia[11] suggested that women and their partners should be given information about the specific purposes of the ultrasound scans and what they can and cannot achieve, so they can be better informed about the limitations of the scans. Some of these sensitive issues are played out to the public on TV, in the news media and on social media, where opinions can vary.

*Adwoa became extremely distressed after the clinician performing the scan told her she could not see her baby's heart clearly. Adwoa had only heard the first part of that statement and thought her baby had died.*

*When Adwoa left space in her distress, the clinician was able to explain that she could hear the heartbeat and see the heart but because of the way the baby was laying, she could not see all four chambers of the heart clearly; and that this was due to the way the baby was lying in the womb.*

*During review with the clinician after Adwoa had left the room, pointing out that had they explained the purpose of this particular scan and what it might reveal could have better prepared the woman to receive any untoward news. Without such preparation such news can be shocking.*

## ISSUES AROUND LOSS AT 22 TO 24 WEEKS: THE THRESHOLD OF VIABILITY

In many countries there are guidelines concerning the gestational age for viability. English law states that 24 weeks is the legal limit for abortions to be undertaken, excluding fatal foetal abnormalities detected after that point. Babies born alive after 22 weeks can and do survive with active resuscitation, mechanical ventilation and other medical interventions but they are subject to possible long-term physical and psychological consequences.

Women who spontaneously go into labour at these gestations face the prospect of the baby dying in labour, at birth or soon after birth. If the baby is born alive, decisions on clinical care will be focused on the likelihood of survival and what that may mean for the family. The parents' wishes and decisions may raise challenges for the professionals giving care.

Statistics about survival at birth can be both informative and confusing; and very distressing for parents to manage in this vulnerable situation. Information from various sources will be used by the teams providing care but as Lynne Gillam[12] states:

> *"Despite the resources and their clinical expertise and experience, clinicians can sometimes struggle to determine which is the best and most ethically appropriate course of action for these babies."*

In these situations, Ali M Nadroo[13] recommends that, "The healthcare team should demonstrate compassion, humility, courage, honesty, sensitivity and commitment, not abandonment."

Some parents have very clear ideas about resuscitation or palliative care that follow their own ethical, religious and moral principles. Others can feel very unprepared and ill-informed to make any decision.

## PROFESSIONAL REACTIONS TO LOSS AT 22-24 WEEKS

Professionals can be offering care to women seeking intended abortion, alongside unwanted loss. Staff are not always supported in the dilemmas they face to give sensitive individualised care. Both the RCOG[14] and the British Association of Perinatal Medicine[14] offer support and guidance in these challenging situations. A consistent team approach offers support whilst the woman, her partner and their family struggle to make sense of the medical options open to them. If their decision is only to offer palliative care at birth and if this tiny baby is born alive, the healthcare professionals can face challenges to their own ethical, moral, social and faith beliefs.

*Sophie had cared for Sinha and Aslam when labour had started at 23 weeks. Their baby was alive with a good heartbeat when Sinha was admitted to the labour ward and, as was usual practice in their Maternity Unit, a senior neonatologist came to see the couple. There was a long conversation concerning the likelihood of the baby being born alive, what could be done to help her to live and her chances for survival, following The British Association of Perinatal Medicine Framework for Clinical Practice at the Time of Birth[14]. Sinha and Aslam had already told Sophie that they would let Allah decide the fate of their baby and nothing the doctors had said changed their decision.*

*Reviewing later the difficult situation in which Sophie found herself, she explained that for her, every life was sacred, and she would have wanted the doctors to give her baby every opportunity to survive, including active resuscitation and neonatal intensive care. She struggled to accept the parents' decision but also wanted to give the care the parents wanted. When the baby was born, she had a very faint, irregular heartbeat but she did not begin breathing. Sinha and Aslam cuddled their little girl and within a few minutes there was no heartbeat. Sophie was very distressed and struggled to manage her feelings. Even though the parents expressed their thanks for respecting their wishes, she found resolving her own conflicts very difficult.*

*In this case, Sophie was applying her own personal value judgements. Whilst talking through this situation in a counselling situation enabled her to express the deeply held beliefs which framed her personal attitude towards saving life, she had not considered what cost and burden this action may have placed on Raiza, Aslam and the little girl.*

*The care she had given was in line with current medical practice, the parents' wishes and the condition of the baby at birth. Her struggle was with the conflict between her personal beliefs and the professional clinical advice.*

# FOLLOW-ON CARE

In the weeks after loss, parents will be grieving and working at making some sense of their experience. Some will be able to make progress by themselves and not feel the need for further contact with any professionals. Others may struggle with questions, worries and anxieties that can take time to frame into words. Other concerns may arise from their experience. The need for follow-up care tailored to their individual needs may not be recognised. Returning to GP care may not offer the information or emotional support they need.

Maintaining contact with a member of the team who cared for them can help in signposting care appropriately and give clients the necessary information and support. Using support networks and information from charities involved with loss may help to answer some questions and to fulfil their needs.

# 4: The Third Trimester: 24 Weeks and Onwards

*Loss before labour; managing labour; during labour; stillbirth occurring in labour; surrogacy and adoption; professionals' reactions to loss in labour; making memories; removal of baby to the mortuary; ceremonies and rituals; decisions about burial or cremation; what happens next; debriefing staff; premature birth; loss of one baby in a multiple pregnancy; neonatal death; maternal death; loss in the wider context; support for the professionals.*

After 23 weeks and six days, a baby is regarded in the UK both clinically and legally to be capable of living outside the mother and, if born at this time, will be supported with all the resuscitation techniques that the neonatal team can employ.

In England and Wales, the stillbirth rate reduced in 2017 to 4.2% per 1000 live and stillbirth ONS[1]. Worldwide WHO[2] figures estimate that 7,000 women experience a stillbirth every day. Pregnancy loss is more prevalent in low and middle-income countries. Globally accurate data collection and standardization differs widely. The WHO is working to "improve data by setting a standardization system for classifying stillbirths and neonatal deaths[3]".

The WHO also collaborated with the UN and several institutions and individual experts to publish 'Every Woman, Every Child', the indicator and monitoring framework for the global strategy for Women's, Children's and Adolescent's Health[4], setting goals to improve standardised data collection which will enable countries to focus on improving health outcomes for women and children.

Headlines and images in the media depict women 'blooming' and happy in this trimester and preparations advance for the baby's arrival. Women wear badges and t-shirts to proclaim their pregnancy. It all becomes very public knowledge. Photographs of the developing bump are shared across media platforms. All these societal expectations can be difficult to live up to.

There are many reasons, not always expressed, why women and their partners feel different to the assumed expectations at this time in the pregnancy. It can be a reaction to the physical changes as her body increases in size and changes shape. The start of this pregnancy may have been unplanned, a shock or unwanted. They now face the reality that their life will change dramatically when this baby is born. Partners may worry that they will lose their special place in their loved one's affections to this baby. Both may suddenly be questioning their abilities as parents.

> Alesha was referred to the counsellor following her 36-week ante-natal midwife visit. At the appointment, she told the midwife that she had expected to feel very happy and excited at this stage of her pregnancy but instead was not looking forward to having her baby and felt that was wrong. With the counsellor, Alesha revealed she felt great ambivalence about becoming a mother. She felt relieved after sharing her worries. In further sessions, she was able to work through issues she had with her own mother, who had died when she was ten. This helped her to understand that the childhood experience of loss was not resolved. Often in pregnancy, deep-seated fears and worries emerge that have been suppressed in order to survive traumatic events.

> At ten, she had had more immediate concerns than considering what becoming a mother would mean for her. Now the absence of her mother was both a loss and a worry for the future. Now she was going to be a mother, would she be confronted with her own mortality? Would history repeat itself? What kind of mother would she be? The loss felt even more acute now and there was no way of finding out how her mother had felt about being pregnant and becoming a mother. All these issues and more came to light and could be acknowledged as she explored the implications of motherhood for herself.

## LOSS BEFORE LABOUR

Women may find out about the death of their baby before it begins during a routine antenatal clinic visit. If the heartbeat cannot be heard, it is usual practice to have an ultrasound scan to confirm the heartbeat has stopped. This either means waiting in a busy clinic with other pregnant women or a very stressful journey to the hospital. Both situations demand sensitive management by the professionals. In a survey undertaken by Jane Arezina[4] at the University of Leeds, radiographers were asked how they learnt to deliver difficult news during a foetal ultrasound examination. The majority (52.6%) had received a lecture-based training from Antenatal Results and Choices (ARC) and a total of 64.9% had received lecture-based, group discussion and role play training. Radiographers play a vital role in delivering antenatal care and can be closely involved in delivering difficult news in their scanning clinics.

Whilst there are guidelines and protocols for training in all areas of healthcare which acknowledge the emotional needs of the client, there are often no clear guidelines for practice, particularly in a pressurised healthcare setting.

Offering information about the next steps helps to support the woman and her partner and helps the professional to feel he/she is giving them something concrete in the midst of all the unknowns. RCOG[6] and NICE[7] both offer clinical guidelines to adopt locally and both touch on the importance of psychological support for women and their families during the processes. NICE has a section on support after traumatic birth, miscarriage or stillbirth.

Doctors, midwives and sonographers find the discussion around the lack of a heartbeat quite difficult. Women recall with great detail how and where they were told and how this is managed will have great influence on how she and her family cope with their loss. This knowledge can intensify the anxiety for the person delivering the information. What to say and what to do is a worry shared by many. Clients are helped by a professional who can look them in the face and use simple short sentences with pauses to allow for them to ask the questions they want to during the conversation. Giving them time to absorb the information enables them to get through the shock. Phrases such as "I can see this is very difficult news to hear" offer empathy. It can also be useful to check what they have understood from the words you have said. This conversation may be more difficult when eye contact is not a part of the cultural norm. Listening to the women and their partners and matching their communication helps the professional to respond authentically and appropriately.

What to say and how to break bad news in difficult situations like those above will be addressed in a future chapter. For the professional, each time is a new and learning experience, and places the individual in an unknown situation. It is never easy. Beate[8] et al recognise there can be personal costs to this caring, which leads to a professional withdrawing from the situation in order to lessen their emotional turmoil. Staff worry about what words to say, how to say them, how to manage the shock at the news, the tears, the explicit displays of grief, their reactions of the woman and her partner, even what danger they may be in if anger is displayed. Some will have developed the words they use out of previous experience. Their behaviour may be defensive if they feel challenged at all. Unexpected dramatic reactions can escalate and disrupt the clinic.

Remaining calm and having the support of another member of the team is important and can help to de-escalate any unwanted situation. Those new to this are often tempted to fill the silence with what they feel is reassuring information. A rush to move the women on from the scan room may show a certain panic about how to manage the situation. This can be met by anger from the woman and she could feel that the professional did not care about her. Silence is necessary, processing both the information and formulating the responses and questions takes time.

Such sensitive information is more difficult to deliver where there are language and/or cultural differences. The use of interpreters via a phone link helps with the practical issues raised. Demonstrating care and concern, whilst maintaining an awareness of the appropriate signals in every situation, may be achieved with eye contact, or even if appropriate, a hand on the shoulder.

*David had been scanning for a year in the antenatal clinic. He had great people skills and was well liked by both his colleagues and the women he scanned. He had worked in the early pregnancy unit so had been involved in giving bad news to women quite often. When he was asked to scan Sarah, who had come to the unit following her midwife appointment at 38 weeks, he thought his experience would help if he had to break bad news. On seeing there was no heartbeat he looked at Sarah to break the news.*

*What he had not expected to see was her reaction. Sarah was white and shocked and hyperventilating and began to shout at him. David was taken off guard but was able to manage the situation and Sarah was introduced to the bereavement midwife for ongoing care. A few days later David was experiencing real anxiety and his open friendly personality changed. This was noticed by his peers. They suggested he talked through this experience with the counsellor.*

*He was very anxious about working in the early pregnancy unit and changed shifts with others to avoid working there. In short, he had lost his confidence in his people skills. Over a couple of sessions, David realised he had not previously been exposed to the reactions Sarah displayed. He had fears about coping with confrontation and anger which he had not addressed and in the counselling space he was able to express his distress about feeling inadequate and ill-equipped. He had not felt that when face-to-face with women in early pregnancy, where loss was more common; but in his own mind this baby was near term and it was different. He had had an emotional response to this loss.*

*He recognised that loss further on in pregnancy was even more unexpected and women may have very different reactions. Women feel much more connected to their baby as he/she develops a character in utero. Not knowing that he/she had died also gives women deep feelings of guilt. How could they not have known? Exploring these and other issues helped him to feel stronger about facing and managing any similar situations.*

In the case of a pregnancy complicated by a known abnormality or a problem pregnancy there is the added stress of potential for death before life or at the beginning of life. For these women and their partners, spending time planning the labour and delivery offers a degree of control over an uncertain future. Discussion around such issues as pain relief and who will be there for the delivery help to focus on what can be normal and to prepare for what will be different. Offering women practical information at the appropriate time is useful and can help staff to feel useful, but only in a framework that also allows for them to discuss fears and worries. Generally, all healthcare staff feel more comfortable in conversations where they can offer practical information and support. The information women want about what happens next demands the staff try to pay attention to the individual's emotional resources.

It is difficult to assess this quickly, but women say that when this news is given in a calm and factual way, it is easier to hear and digest the information. This often needs to be repeated and given in written form which can be locally produced to provide procedures and support contacts. There is useful research on how information is given and the effect that has on understanding, memory compliance and satisfaction, which we will reflect on in a later chapter.

There are often tears and shock at the news that labour will be induced medically not only from the woman but also from her close family and friends. Whilst Cingi[9] *et al* state that the manner in which the information is communicated can be just as important as the information being conveyed. The language we use at this time also affects the woman and her capacity to negotiate through her loss. Using words and simple phrases in non-technical language will aid effective communication. Also, checking understanding along the way helps to ensure women are fully aware of what is happening.

How much more difficult this becomes in the presence of both language and cultural differences. Professional interpreters will be aware of the need to make sure women understand all the information they need to know and give the opportunity for questions.

Women will often challenge the medical induction of labour process. At this point going through labour can seem an added insult to them. Often partners and family will ask "can't she just be put to sleep and have a caesarean?" It is at the moment accepted that inducing a vaginal birth when labour has not started is considered safer but the questioning by the woman and her family can be difficult to handle. Explaining the reasons, which are to do with her safety and recovery, and taking the time to address the questions that arise, helps to resolve worries and concerns.

## MANAGING LABOUR

Medical induction of labour is a two-step process and during the few days before the woman is admitted, there is time for the reality about the death of her baby to really sink in. Openness and honesty are the cornerstones of the relationship through this difficult time. Questions at this time are often centred around, "Why did this happen to me?". There may be no answers to give and stating the reality of, "We don't know" seems inadequate.

Phrases that can help include, "The reasons for your baby dying at this stage are not always known", "There are investigations and tests that can be done" and "We will share all the results we have with you but it may take time". This may feel inadequate for the professional but if the woman feels the approach is genuine, she is more likely to understand and accept this information

Where this can be done, devising and recording a birth plan all help to settle the mind about labour. Writing this down enhances the opportunity for effective communication, as there will often be different health professionals involved when labour starts.

*Hannah had been fully informed about the heart condition diagnosed for her son. She knew this meant he may not survive labour and birth. She had many appointments for scans and met the paediatric team who would be caring for him, even visiting the unit to which he would be transferred. What was not covered in these consultations was how she could be supported in labour. Hannah spent time with the midwife counsellor talking about her feelings about what was already an unknown experience. This was her first baby and the added stress of not knowing whether her son would be born alive or not. When Hannah had met the doctors who would care for her baby, they had discussed what might happen if he was born alive.*

*It appeared that her way of coping and managing the stress associated with the unknown was to research the condition her baby had as fully as she could and question the doctors in detail on points about which she was uncertain. This can feel like a challenge to the professionals but is just the struggle to have some control in uncertain circumstances. She felt alone through all this as her partner was finding thinking about his son needing surgical intervention very soon after his birth traumatic, so was avoiding addressing this with her or anyone else.*

*There were other questions about how much control she had in these distressing circumstances. She wanted a normal labour and would have asked for a home delivery. Already, there were losses she had experienced, with more to come. The loss of control over where her labour took place, being induced, decisions about having labour augmented to put as little pressure on the baby as possible all seemed to make sense for the baby but Hannah was feeling quite left out of these decisions and was unable to voice her concerns for herself. The professionals seemed to concentrate on the best management for her son and her needs were not even being voiced. When what was expected turns into a series of previously unknown challenges, our own sense of what is certain in our world is cast out and Hannah had been left to manage this by herself. She was fearful about raising some of these issues with the professionals, as she felt they may think her needs were not as important as those of her son.*

*It was only after her referral to the counsellor that she had the space to have her worries and concerns heard. When picking up this issue in the clinic situation, where other constraints are on the professional, it can be difficult to tune into and pick up on underlying, unperceived problems.*

*The doctor who suggested she came to see the counsellor was concerned as she appeared very anxious but had not known specifically what it was about. This may often be the case when doctors, midwives or sonographers refer to the counsellor. Issues can be uncovered within the work of the counselling that can significantly change the psychological outcome for both the woman and the team caring for her. Helping Hannah to put herself back in the decision process enabled her to give voice to her needs both with the doctors and her partner. This helped her partner to feel a part of this pregnancy again. Together with the team, they agreed plans for her labour that included Hannah in the decision-making process.*

## DURING LABOUR

When care is being given after pregnancy loss, the labour room takes on a different tone. The focus and excitement of greeting this baby is gone, replaced by the sadness of loss and often anxiety about how the baby will look. If there are known abnormalities, women can be anxious about their reactions but even in the worst of circumstances, carefully preparing both baby and family can lead to creating memories that focus on normality: perhaps the perfectly normal hands, feet or face.

Asking the woman and her partner before the birth how *they* want to see the baby puts them in control. Here again, paying attention to the woman's religious and cultural background and, if not known, establishing her wishes, signifies a caring approach.

There is only one opportunity to get this right and not knowing all the nuances can prevent staff from giving the appropriate care. If there are religious staff attached to the hospital, they can be a valuable resource of information for staff, women and their families, who may be confused about their faith rites.

Finding the words to say to women and their families at this time causes all healthcare professionals anxiety. Offering words such as, "I am so sorry this is happening/has happened to you" recognises their distressing experience, whilst distancing the event from the person. In other words, empathy not sympathy. Another phrase which helps at this time is, "We are here to be with you through this". This phrase helps to connect with the woman and her family and to create a space where they can share concerns and ask questions throughout what can be a very lonely experience.

The skill and art of the midwife is much needed by the family and at this time empathy, patience and encouragement can help to settle them. This is a demanding role and support by other members of the team can be of great assistance. Practical support, such as offering to prepare the cot for the baby or completing some of the paperwork, demonstrates a caring support team and makes a tough situation slightly easier. SANDS UK is a resource used by many UK hospitals which offers training and support to all professionals with the practical aspects of bereavement care. This includes the paperwork based on best practice and current research, and checklists to aid in the provision of care.

The labour ward can be a busy, loud place. It is useful to talk about this with the family who will be walking in and out of the labour room. Best practice is to have separate entrances and exits but this is often not practical in the labour suites. It is important that all staff on shift are aware of the situation in order to maintain privacy for the family, and so that no-one unknowingly says something inappropriate.

## STILLBIRTH OCCURRING IN LABOUR

An unexpected stillbirth during labour is shocking for all involved and by its nature, there is little opportunity for preparation. It is less common and may relate to decision-making in labour. The team caring for the woman will be shocked but must continue to offer appropriate care. They will operate on an action level and only after the situation do they allow their feelings to emerge. Nuzum[10] et al undertook semi-structured interviews of eight obstetric and gynaecology consultants in Ireland. This is a small sample but it highlights the lack of knowledge available on how the experience impacts on professionals. They encountered displays of emotion when the interviewees talked about their experience of caring during stillbirth. None of the doctors had had any training in how best to deal with this situation. All had experienced many emotions and had found no support in managing their feelings. They also highlighted the issues of medico-legal concerns that may have impacted on the care they offered.

Professionals can feel anxious about displaying emotions whilst caring for a bereaved woman. Wallbank[11] and Begley[12] both recount stories from midwives, nurses and student midwives who cried with women, demonstrating how much they emotionally attach to the experience.

## SURROGACY AND ADOPTION

Loss will also be a factor to consider when caring for the birth mother and her family, when babies are given to the intended parents after birth through surrogacy arrangements. When a baby is to be given into foster care or straight for adoption, the birth mother may well exhibit many emotions, including loss and grief. In both circumstances, women may want to be discharged early from the hospital environment, but they deserve the opportunity to have their feelings valued and discussed in the postnatal period.

This can be challenging for the professional but recognising that this is not an easy loss to experience and recover from, whether through choice or circumstance, goes a long way to support through very unusual life events. It is more important to focus on giving supportive emotional care to those in need than to understand the motivations for these decisions.

## PROFESSIONALS' REACTIONS TO LOSS IN LABOUR

*Following a very difficult forceps delivery, the midwife who was caring for the woman continued to offer excellent care and undertook all the tasks she was required to do until the end of her shift. Shock only set in when she went home and the tears began to flow. She was not scheduled to work for a couple of days and hoped that she would feel a little better and be able to return to work. When she walked on to the delivery suite again, she started shaking and again was in tears*

*The labour ward was busy but the coordinator realised that the midwife would not be able to work without some support and so contacted the bereavement midwife to ask her to offer a space to talk and support. The bereavement midwife offered active listening, a non-judgemental space and private time. This helped the midwife to let out her feelings, have her distress acknowledged, and to have a safe space in which to reveal her anxieties.*

*This was separate and different to the multidisciplinary review of the processes involved but it enabled the midwife to be clear about her role in the labour and prepared for the management intervention which happens after untoward and unexpected incidents. Building in resilience for staff at all levels could benefit the service.*

## MAKING MEMORIES

Many years ago, women who suffered a stillbirth were given no opportunity to see or cuddle their baby and were offered no memory items such as a lock of hair or a name band. Working as a bereavement midwife, I received letters from women who had a stillbirth 30-40 years ago and who wrote eloquently about their continuing sadness at not seeing their baby and the ever-present loss they felt. They asked if their baby had had a funeral. What had happened to the body?

Over the past twenty years, this has all changed and women's wishes are now taken into account when considering whether to see or hold their baby, to take photos, add any memory tokens they wish to have to lovingly created memory boxes; and to make their own funeral plans, all supported and guided by their carers. Maternity Units have supplies of clothes and memory items and boxes available to choose from and some use professional photographers for family photos. Penny Hughes[13] *et al* set out to assess if holding their dead infant had measurable psychological benefits for women and amongst their findings, they concluded that those who had held their baby were more likely to suffer from depression than those who just saw their baby; and those who did not see their baby were less likely to become depressed. Other variables, such as holding a funeral and keeping memory items, did not appear to have any untoward outcomes. Following this paper, advice in the UK is to offer physical contact after birth but also to respect those who decline this offer.

In Sweden, a paper published by Kerstin Eriandsson[14] *et al* reviewed the experiences of mothers after their stillbirth and saw a trend towards something they termed "assumptive bonding", which they saw as the carer presenting the baby to the mother in a simple and natural way. This seemed to be an acceptable practice. There is no right or wrong way to manage this situation but starting the conversation and framing the questions around what would be acceptable to the woman and her partner helps the caregiver to act compassionately, sensitively and in accordance with their clients' wishes. There is value in also acknowledging that they can change their mind at any time.

## REMOVAL OF A BABY TO THE MORTUARY

This can be a traumatic event. Saying goodbye is never easy. It reinforces loss. A useful way of introducing this subject is when the healthcare provider is asked, "What happens next?". The parents can then be given the opportunity to prepare themselves a little for saying goodbye in a way that is under their control. Individual hospital arrangements will be in place for taking the baby out of the hospital. Women may want to take their baby home for a brief time and local hospitals will have their own procedures to follow.

## CEREMONIES AND RITUALS AFTER DEATH

Most religions and cultures will have a ceremony that pays respect in a mosque, synagogue or church. Crematoriums and Cemeteries also provide chapels for those who mourn to have some time to say a public goodbye before burial or cremation. Contact with those who can officiate can be offered and they will help arrangements can be made before leaving the hospital.

## DECISIONS ABOUT BURIAL OR CREMATION

Decisions about burial or cremation may be based on cultural and religious practices but again, the opportunity to learn what choices are available enables decisions to be made that may differ from cultural norms. The speed with which the service happens is time critical to those of the Jewish and Muslim beliefs. If a post-mortem is decided upon, then burial or cremation may have to be delayed. This issue can cause conflict between the families and the medical personnel. Some families will not consent to post-mortem for the above reasons. Mortuaries that undertake post-mortems for babies are aware of these issues and will try to accommodate the wishes of the parents where they can. Local Chaplains, used to dealing with both, can be very helpful in resolving these issues and if there are questions that need further explanation, they can offer non-judgmental support to those in need.

### WHAT HAPPENS NEXT?

Women want and need to know that their tragedy matters to the professionals. Explaining to them the process of investigation that follows a stillbirth helps them to feel their loss is attended to; and so it is important for the professionals to explain each step that is taken in the review the hospital undertakes that works towards an understanding of how this could have happened and if there are reasons why this has happened. Over the last few years, professionals have become more accessible and best practice is to keep the parents involved throughout the next weeks by establishing a point of contact and encouraging open contact when required.

## DEBRIEFING STAFF AFTER LOSS

Much work has been published about the value of debriefing for staff involved in critical incidents. Hospital emergency units have set up systems for a debriefing which facilitates "...discussion of actions and thought processes, encourage reflection, and ultimately assimilate improved behaviours into practice[15]". This recognises there is value in both giving space for ventilation of feelings and reflection. The timing and content of these meetings may be overseen by management and may concentrate more on the events that happened, which can also inform the feedback for families involved in the incident. Staff tensions can be addressed in these sessions. There is value in having a strong lead, so that it benefits each person in the group. Blame is not the focus and ventilation of emotions about the situation is allowed. The emphasis on learning from the situation is valuable but may expose deficits in the person and/or in the system, leaving feelings of vulnerability and exposure. Multidisciplinary reviews focus on the facts of the events but local informal debriefing among the staff directly involved allows for expression of emotions and signposts support for those who want it. Wallbank and Richardson[11] explored midwifery and nursing staffs' responses to miscarriage, stillbirth and neonatal loss, and some of their conclusions highlighted the need for training which normalises the emotional responses to loss with supportive interventions for all staff, enabling those who do not feel confident in delivering care to address and overcome their anxieties and so spread the load amongst their peers.

Midwives in the UK have benefitted from supervisors who offered a reflective space separate to the management process. Here, midwives had the opportunity to express their emotions and anxieties following any distressing event they have experienced or been involved with and this has been a valuable source of support.

Other professionals may not have access to support and often employ different coping strategies. Contact with the women and their families may not be as intimate and constant as the midwife. Is it safe to assume that because they don't share or talk about their feelings associated with loss that their coping strategies help them? Or are they in denial? They may allow an objectivity whilst they focus on the medical issues. Asking these questions even silently may give insight and enable support to be offered.

## PREMATURE BIRTH

In 2016, the stillbirth rate for babies born at 24 weeks gestation was 356.4 stillbirths per 1,000 total births. This compares with a rate of 1.2 at 40 weeks' gestation ONS[1].

The loss of expectations of normality can lead to feelings of failure when a baby is born prematurely. With a baby on the edge of life and death, there is also the continuing fear of impending loss. This may not be actual death, but women are fearful of hearing bad news about the health of their baby alongside the risks of physical and mental impairment. Loss is also connected to their dreamed of perfect child. There can also be family stresses, other children, and fears for the future that complicate the process of grieving

> *Lily was born at 26 weeks following a short labour. Her mother June was very shocked after the birth and staff reported that she did not seem to want to visit her baby, concentrating on arrangements for the care of her other children. June was fit*

*and there was no medical reason for her to stay in the maternity unit, so she went home. The community midwives and the staff in the neonatal unit were also concerned about June as she was not coming in to see her baby. Finding the opportunity to talk with June was not easy. When Lily became ill, June did visit her and the staff were able to begin the conversation about her feelings about Lily.*

*June was very frightened after the birth of Lily. She feared that she would die and so disengaged herself to avoid the pain of loss. She thought that if she did not "bond" with her then she would "get over it" more quickly. It was the fear of actual loss when Lily became ill that brought her back to the Unit.*

*June had complex social problems and did not engage with professionals well, which led her to avoid talking to the staff. She was worried about sharing personal information and so was holding back. This had become a bewildering situation for her, and she was dealing with it in the only way she knew how.*

*It took a few sessions for June to feel comfortable with discussing her feelings and a non-judgmental approach allowed her to start to let the counsellor hear her sadness, guilt, anger. When those feelings were released, June owned them and was able to cry for the first time.*

This intervention used the counselling principles of active listening and validation of feelings of the actual loss and fear about the impending loss.

## LOSS OF ONE BABY IN A MULTIPLE PREGNANCY

The loss of one baby of a multiple pregnancy can occur at any time in utero: at birth when one baby is stillborn; and into the neo-natal period when one of the babies dies. In a report for MBBRACE – UK, Draper[16] et al report a significant reduction in both the stillbirth and neonatal death rate ratios associated with twin pregnancies over the period 2014 to 2016, to 1.6 % for stillbirths and 3.33% for neonatal deaths.

If early loss of one twin is seen on a scan after a positive diagnosis of a twin pregnancy the term "vanishing twin" is used. Later loss in the second and third trimester may result in the non-viable twin becoming mummified in utero, which is known as "foetus papyraceous". This can be seen on scan during the pregnancy and may be evident at birth. If this is seen in a monochorionic twin pregnancy, then the risks are higher to the other twin and monitoring for the living twin will increase. The woman and her partner will need information and support during pregnancy and, following delivery, help with making decisions about funeral options.

When a death happens in a multiple pregnancy, delight gives way to despair, then feelings of guilt can set in when there is a baby still alive. There is inevitably huge conflict in managing death and life at the same time.

If the birth has been premature then the potential added complication of babies being transferred to different hospitals depending on their needs adds to the conflict. These and other issues complicate and affects the course of the grief process for mother and father and the wider family. Many may focus on the surviving baby to avoid the loss but there is no comfort to be had from loose comments such as, "Well, at least you have one baby". Sadly, this has been said by healthcare professionals as well as family members. It may be that they truly think this situation has compensations and that this can help lessen the loss! In fact, it can make the situation very much worse for the family as it emphasises the conflict the mother is already feeling.

Both mother and father will feel loss of being parents to more than one baby. They worry that grieving affects their ability to care for or be interested in the surviving baby. There is an overwhelming fear that this baby, too, could become ill or die. Professionals can help the woman and her family by explaining that whilst these feelings are very uncomfortable and frightening, these are normal reactions in these circumstances. Emotional support may need to continue long after discharge, as the parents cope with the registration and funeral process. Anxiety about the living twin will continue well into the first year and beyond. Wellness checks with either GP or neonatal consultant will give practical support. Research into the experience of mothers who suffered a loss of one twin was published by Judy Richards[17] *et al.* They interviewed 14 mothers who had suffered the loss of one baby in pregnancy or in the neo-natal period and found that many women delay their grief, or "put it on hold", so that they can support the other baby. How long this goes on for is not known as the research has not been done yet.

Nancy Segal[18] from the Twinless Twins Support Group International, points to the effect on the surviving twin which is seen to pursue them into adulthood. Survivor guilt may be a factor and parents can be introduced to this at an appropriate time so that they are prepared for this possibility. Segal recommends further research on this topic.

Since the advent of multiple conceptions relating to fertility treatments and the offer of selective termination, the emotional sequelae on women and their surviving children when selective termination is used would also benefit from further specific research to help support those who choose this form of management in their pregnancy. NICE published the Multiple pregnancy: antenatal care for twin and triplet pregnancies clinical guideline[19] to help reduce the incidence of loss but does not address the emotional needs of families after loss. Richards[17] concludes that there are specific emotional issues faced by mothers after the loss of one baby and that there is more to discover about their particular needs.

TAMBA, the twins and multiple births association, undertake research and offer support for women, their partners and families through all experiences. For information and support, the Multiple Births Foundation is a charity concerned with all issues around multiple pregnancies and births.

## NEONATAL DEATH

The teams caring for premature and sick babies, whilst managing the long-term care of these babies, may be faced with preparing for their death. There may be very difficult conversations to be had with parents. These conversations require very sensitive approaches and may conflict with the desires of the parents to continue care. The professionals involved are making decisions about how, when and what to share with the parents and who gets to be involved in making the decision about turning off the ventilator when the medical opinion is that death is inevitable. The long-term consequences for the parents and their individual circumstances directs the professionals in their approach. Parents may be interacting with other parents in special care/intensive care where they get some support but also shared anxiety and sometimes misinformation. They are often comparing the health and treatment of their own and other babies.

*Sally was born prematurely at 28 weeks after her mother, Maggie, came to the labour ward with an antepartum haemorrhage. She was in a very poor condition and resuscitated at birth and taken to the neo-natal unit where she was ventilated. There was concern immediately for her and the decision was made to transfer her to another intensive unit. This was a difficult situation for Maggie and her partner, already reeling from the shock of the events that had led to her birth. Maggie could not at that point travel with her so there was much pain at the separation. Over the next few days, Maggie became well but sadly, Sally developed an overwhelming infection and died when she was four days old. Maggie had by this time been transferred to be with her daughter and was discharged home from there.*

*The community midwife visiting the family recognised that they had many psychological needs. She felt that at some point they could benefit from counselling and contacted the Bereavement Midwife for advice and for her to make contact with the family. At this time, neither Maggie nor her partner felt able to talk but they contacted the Bereavement Counsellor six weeks later.*

*Both parents had differing needs and they were feeling miles apart from each other in their grieving. Her partner was feeling very angry and was not sure how to deal with this within their relationship. Maggie was not feeling connected to her life. She spent a lot of the day just looking into space and avoiding the difficult feelings she had. In the sessions they benefited from having a safe space to vent their feelings. They had felt unable to talk about their feelings with each other for fear of upsetting their partner. The role of the counsellor in this situation is to be a listening ear for them both. In this space couples can listen and truly hear the other person and their distress as they talk to the counsellor.*

*Maggie's partner was feeling rejected by his wife who appeared to resist any suggestions he was making about helping her to manage her grief. Maggie felt alone with her loss and even more so after the funeral, as friends and relations returned to their normal lives.*

*Exploring their different approaches to their loss and acknowledging that both responses to loss were normal gave them both relief. They began to talk more and recognised that the spaces they occupied were different but not exclusive, as under these reactions were commonalities. They came to recognise each other's needs and felt encouraged to talk more to each other and listen to and accept their differences.*

There can be pressure about the timing of and need for counselling very early on after loss. This is often born out of a genuine need to offer something to help someone to 'feel better'. Women often don't have the words to use to express their deep distress soon after their loss. It is valuable to give information to women and their loved ones about what they can expect to feel in the grieving process. Even explaining the possible reactions presents some normality and helps them not to worry if they experience some or all of them.

There is much information on social media that can be useful, and women can seek out what they need to support them. Most of what can be found on the web is about grief in general, but this may be all that is required. This is a time when women may turn to their GP for support. There is value in watchful waiting for some time, to see how the individual is managing and stepping in with the offer of counselling when distress appears to be increasing rather than resolving. There is no 'best time'. It will depend on the individual and the work of counselling can be more useful when the individual feels able to engage with another person to discuss her feelings.

The loss of any child has consequences for all the family and other children. Women worry about what to tell their children and how to tell them this event they were looking forward to is not going to happen. Making decisions about the child/children meeting their brother/sister can be very challenging and divisive to the family. Taking through this can be challenging for staff too. Remembering that it is the family who have to learn to live with this major crisis can help to focus on the individual needs within the family and allow for non-judgmental support. SANDS have developed leaflets for family members which support them and offer information on how best to support the immediate family. Finding long-term emotional support for struggling families will depend on the local availability of counselling services. There are charities set up to manage these gaps and searching for them locally and offering their contact encourages families to reach out.

## MATERNAL DEATH

The tragedy of a maternal death is a shattering experience for the family and also reverberates through the maternity unit and seriously affects the professional individuals involved. The surveillance of all maternal deaths in the UK is undertaken by MBRRACE (Mothers and Babies: Reducing Risk through Audits and Confidential Enquiries across the UK). In their last report, published in 2018[20], they reported "a five-fold difference (increase) in maternal mortality rates amongst women from Black ethnic backgrounds and an almost twofold difference (increase) amongst women from Asian Ethnic backgrounds, compared to white women." Overall in 2014-16, "9.8 women per 100,000 died during pregnancy or up to six weeks after childbirth or the end of pregnancy. Most women who died had multiple health problems or other vulnerabilities."

Death may happen before labour and be unconnected to the pregnancy. It can be in labour or as a complication of a maternal medical condition. The cause will most likely be ill-defined until the results of the post-mortem are confirmed by the coroner. For women who die after birth, there are both physical and mental health issues. In the UK, a post-mortem is a requirement after a maternal death and may add to the emotional distress of the family if they have conflicting ethical and cultural views about post-mortem examination.

Shock often renders humans speechless and both the family and the professionals involved will struggle to find words to say. For those who either do not speak English or do not use English as their first language, conveying complex information can test the communication skills of the professionals in very extreme circumstances.

It is not possible to prepare for breaking this awful news. Whilst words may not convey the distress felt by the team, the physical demeanour of the professionals will speak a thousand words. Making eye contact with the next of kin is important and what is said will depend on the prior conversations undertaken. Phrases such as, "I am so sorry to be breaking this news" and, "Despite all our interventions, we have been unable to save the life of......." are helpful. Using the correct name is very important to make families feel that the staff are really engaged.

These words will be devastating to hear, so reactions may be startling. It is wise to ensure there is both another professional in the room and support for the next of kin. Care may be given in other places than the maternity department, which can complicate communications and cause further distress. Wherever and whenever, it is, it is unexpected and shocking.

The relationships with the woman who has died and her family will be at different levels for the members of staff involved. Those less engaged with the processes that led to the death may find it easier to talk to the family, and identifying a link person used to negotiating through loss gives the family a familiar contact.

In a report for the Royal College of Midwives, Rosemary Mander[21] interviewed 32 midwives with experience of caring for a mother who died. Amongst her conclusions, she signposted the difficulty encountered by the midwives to separate the professional role from their personal life. This can have serious consequences for the individual involved and underlines that these issues must be taken into account by managers when considering pastoral care in these circumstances.

> *Sara was in ITU after being admitted from home at 26-weeks with little positive signs of life. She was resuscitated but her baby had died and she was on life support. The family had pulled together and there was 24-hour support and contact with them as they took it in turns to sit by her bedside the midwifery team continued to give care and help Toreg, her husband, through the minefield of managing the loss of his baby.*

*Two days later, tests were done to determine the extent of the brain stem injury and they concluded that Sara had no signs of life and they wanted to withdraw all support. The family were attending daily meetings with the team caring for Sara and knew the tests were being done. Toreg had been very quiet, as could be expected from his northern European heritage, but he asked what he needed to know. Sara's sister behaved very differently and questioned loudly every procedure that her sister was undergoing and had demonstrated anger toward the professionals.*

*There was an opportunity to both prepare the room for the conversation and the attendees and they had time together before Toreg, Sara's sister and mother came into the room. The Consultant, whom they knew talked about the tests that were undertaken and explained the results, what they meant and they were asking the family to allow them to withdraw life support. Immediately Sara's sister threw herself onto the floor and grabbed the hand of the consultant pleading with him for this not to be true. Whilst Toreg appeared to withdraw into himself as he shrunk back into a corner where he was sitting. The nurse present reached for Sara's sister but she resisted being moved. The counsellor gently asked the professionals to give her a few minutes and slowly she got up and went to Toreg and he put his arms around her whilst they cried together.*

Such displays of emotions can be devastating for the professionals too. There is a feeling of wanting to make it better and to find solutions, but it does not quite ring true in the face of this particular circumstance. Coping mechanisms may not initially engage, as these situations are very rare and unusual. The degree of emotional involvement with the family can also dictate the response. The ITU team have experience of these life and death situations and will have more developed professional and personal coping mechanisms.

Generally, the greater the person employs emotional distance, the more able they seem to be able to cope. Midwives work carefully to develop close relationships with women and their families, so they often do not have this distance and these shattering events have serious consequences which include high death anxiety mild to moderate death obsession and mild death depression. Muliira[22]. Seeking help and support can be seen as a failure to cope, so those needs can be denied and suppressed until the next time they are caring through any trauma. Others around them can help by recognising their needs and working with them to find the help they need. This may be within the profession or hospital or through their GP or other counselling agencies.

Ongoing support for the family may be delivered by the management team. The same team will be involved in the practical information gathering and reporting which will proceed to local investigation in the first instance; then wider involvement in investigation and a potential coroner's hearing. To expect this team to offer appropriate emotional support has not been fully explored in the NHS and may not fit comfortably with the family. Their anger can push the team into a defensive stance and block open conversations where issues of care can be voiced. Those who are familiar with what happens after death could be best placed to offer practical support and information. This may be the Midwifery bereavement team or the chaplains in the hospital. The long-term emotional needs of the family will be complex and requires services outside the hospital and include such charities such as CRUSE.

When considering the emotional needs of the partner and other children in the family, Zhu[23] et al found that surviving children were more likely to have difficulties with their studies culminating with dropping out of school. Husbands had poor mental health and a high incidence of PTSD.

To date there is no formal structure within all units that offers confidential support services and/or debriefing facilities to either families or staff involved in a maternal death. This may change if the Bereavement Care pathway still in development is adopted at all hospitals in England nbcpathway.org.uk.

## LOSS IN THE WIDER CONTEXT

At this point, it is important to reflect that loss without death is experienced in many different ways throughout the pregnancy journey. The loss of the perfect child when abnormalities are diagnosed or a labour does not progress as expected, meaning medical and surgical interventions to expedite delivery; when there is cause for concern for either mother, baby or both, and when there is the loss of the planned for perfect labour and delivery.

Emergencies are expected and prepared for by the professionals but the experience for the woman and her family is very different. Whilst safety is vital, recognising the psychological and emotional needs of the woman and her partner and family are often forgotten.

Amongst the team, one person should reach out to the waiting family to explain the emergency in simple terms and to ensure they have somewhere appropriate to wait. The feelings of relief when both mother and baby are safe can mask and put on hold the feelings that were experienced but they often surface later. The offer of support and counselling can be repeated after the event has resolved.

*Katy sat hugging her daughter as tears fell down from her eyes. She looked exhausted and said she was not sleeping much at all. Her daughter seemed oblivious to the distress her mother was feeling as she slept peacefully. Katy was finding placing her in the cot difficult, her husband was back at work and she had no relatives close to support her. Whilst this may be something many new mums experience, Katy had had a labour she did not expect. It took some time for Katy to raise her feelings about her labour. She said she was trying to put it behind her but when she did get some sleep she was waking up in panic and sometimes sweating and shaking.*

*There were parts of her labour she did not want to recall but she felt understanding what had actually happened may help her find some of the control she felt she had lost. I suggested one way to do this would be to go through her records together when she felt able and wanted to. This seemed to help settle her for a while. Two weeks later, she called for another appointment. We had decided together to undertake this session at her home and she wanted her partner present too.*

*Even seeing the written notes caused her some anxiety but we began by focusing on what was normal through her pregnancy and at the start of her labour. Katy and her partner were encouraged to talk about what went well through that time. I was confirming at each stage that they were comfortable to progress through the more challenging part of her labour. The notes stated the facts and some of the events of the emergency which were agreed by the couple. Technical questions that were raised could not all be answered but were noted so that they could be addressed with the doctor at the consultant follow up meeting.*

*Katy and her partner both wept as they allowed the fears to emerge. She was frightened that their daughter would die and would have done anything that was needed at that time. Whilst trying to be reassuring to her he had been very frightened that he could lose them both and there was no one supporting his needs. He knew she was taken to theatre and he could not be with her. This increased his worry and he went out of the labour ward, sat in his car and cried. Coming back in was very scary and he had to ask where she was and what was happening. This session was the first time either of them had voiced some of their fears to each other and they sat for quite a while holding each other.*

*The session proved to be a turning point for them both as a couple and as new parents. Being able to share their worries with each other helped them to realise they had the support each of them needed.*

As illustrated in the above story, some women do need to have the opportunity to talk about their birth experiences with a professional. Sharing thoughts and feelings can enable better communications between partners too. Responding effectively to the woman's needs demands we help women to review and understand the processes that led to the birth so that they can finish their journey[24]. Interventions may sometimes be led by an obstetrician or a neonatologist, depending on the information required.

A Cochrane review by Bastos[25] *et al* of research into the value of offering psychological care through de-briefing for women following any difficult birth did not find supportive evidence that routine de-briefing made any difference to preventing psychological trauma. It suggested further good quality research to validate these results. Many authors have written about de-briefing in the postnatal period amongst them are Collins[24], Ayers[26], Rowan[27], Kersting[28], Gold[29], Huberty[30]. They all have differing views on what is offered, where it is undertaken and what is the best time for women to receive this service.

## SUPPORT FOR THE PROFESSIONALS

Anyone who is present at traumatic situations will have their own professional and personal reactions. Some will have coping mechanisms that allow them to manage their emotional reactions. After any event the team benefit from an approach which offers them time in a safe place to discuss their emotional reactions and needs. In the UK, the Health and Safety Executive[31] have published a guide to providing support for staff after an incident which comprehensively sets out the potential consequences on the individual and points to how to manage the aftermath in any setting.

# 5: Mental Health

*Mental health in pregnancy; mental health and the professionals; depression; treatment of depression; OCD; anxiety; general anxiety disorder; PTSD; treatment of GAD and PTSD; eating disorders; psychosis; treatment of psychosis; drug and alcohol misuse; health professionals and the care of patients with mental health problems; mental health of the professionals; access to mental health care.*

Mental health problems can affect women and their partners at any stage in pregnancy and post-partum; and can vary from low mood, anxiety and depression to psychotic episodes. A small study in South East London by Howard[1] found that when interviewed with a diagnostic gold standard, one in four pregnant and postpartum women had a mental illness.

Loss in pregnancy and the post-partum period increases the risk of mental health problems, especially for those women who have already suffered some illness. Mental health disorders can be divided into five, sometimes overlapping, areas. These are: a) psychological distress, that is stress and burnout; b) common disorders including depression and anxiety; c) severe disorders such as schizophrenia and bipolar affective disorder; d) cognitive impairment, dementia or the secondary effects of depression and e) substance dependence and the misuse of substances. The charity MIND in the UK has a clear website describing these conditions their diagnosis and treatment.

## MENTAL HEALTH IN PREGNANCY

Pregnant and postpartum women are vulnerable to the same mental health conditions as at other times of their life. The WHO figures suggest about 9% suffering from common disorders such as depression and anxiety. There are some particular features of the pregnancy and postpartum periods that may be different and may affect their mental health adversely. The normal anxiety associated with a change in life may be increased in some women, as may the changes in their body shape. They may be unwilling to tell anyone about their feelings because they are concerned about being stigmatised, of information being recorded in their notes, or even that they might lose custody of the baby. Those taking medication may stop taking their tablets, fearful of the effect on the foetus. This must be checked with them and they should be encouraged to discuss it with their prescriber.

Intervention is also more urgent at this time to manage the effects on the mother but also the foetus and those close to her. We will see that bipolar disorder has an increased risk of recurrence in pregnancy. There is no evidence that other pre-existing mental health problems are particularly altered by pregnancy itself[2], but loss in pregnancy and the immediate postpartum period may increase the likelihood of PTSD, a depressive or anxious reaction, or self-medicating with drugs or alcohol.

## MENTAL HEALTH AND THE PROFESSIONALS

An awareness of the mental health conditions that may be encountered is vital for health professionals working with pregnant mothers and their newborns. The Royal College of Midwives recommends that "all maternity professionals should be equally concerned with mental as well as physical health in pregnancy, childbearing and the postnatal period". Information about mental health is available in the UK from the NHS website, as well as charities such as MIND.

Dealing with mental health issues in the pregnant and postpartum woman requires both assessment of her mental health state and knowledge of access to treatment if required. It can be difficult to assess changes in mental state as many of the indicators we would check for at any other time, may be "normal" at this time. Things such as sleep disturbance, appetite changes, tiredness and loss of libido, general anxiety about the baby and how to manage are normal in pregnancy. It may require a careful clinical assessment to recognise a mental health problem.

It may also not be possible to access a history of the mother's mental health, so empathetic questioning is important. She will be able to tell you everything you need to know if she feels safe in giving you the information, that she is not being judged and understands why you need to know. Not every woman will feel safe enough and that may relate to her past experiences. Women who have been abused or trafficked may feel unable to speak about those experiences.

If healthcare staff pick up a sense that the client seems fearful and reticent, it may only be possible to signpost areas of help. Some clients may feel that the situation is too public or too rushed. It may not be possible to get around this in a busy clinic but if the woman, and sometimes her partner, feel there is someone they can talk to in a safe, private space, it may be enough to reassure them. There are NICE guidelines for the care of Antenatal and Postnatal Mental Health. These reflect programmes that identify and prevent perinatal mood disorders. They cover the treatment of mental health problems in women during pregnancy and the postnatal period up to one year after childbirth. They also provide preconception advice for women with mental health problems and information on the organisation of services in pregnancy and the postnatal period.

The World Health Organization publishes objectives regarding maternal mental health. These include providing support to member states on evidence-based, cost effective and human rights oriented mental health and social care; providing strategies for the promotion of psychosocial well-being; and the prevention of mental disorders in pregnancy and after delivery. They also intend to strengthen information systems, evidence and relevant research.

Mental Health America in 2013 adopted a policy and practice guidelines after concerns about what they consider to be the high rate of infant mortality and medical care not meeting the needs of parents. They suggest screening for perinatal mood and anxiety disorders with follow-up care if required as part of treatment and care plans. Mental health professionals should be located in the settings where the screening is undertaken, in order to offer immediate evaluation, support and diagnosis. The MHA paper suggests increased education about mental health alongside screening and encouraging employers to have occupational health support for pregnant women.

In the study by Howard[1] referred to above, depression was found to be a problem in 11%, anxiety in 15%, eating disorders in 2% of the women studied and 2% were found to be suffering from PTSD. A large study in GP practices in Bradford, England by Prady[3] et al found that the estimated general population figures of about 9% for common mental health disorders rose to about 14% three years postnatally. The study found that between 31.3% and 46.8% were potentially missed in general practice and that minority ethnic women were twice as likely to have potentially missed common mental disorders. The authors suggest that there may be a lack of culturally validated and non-English speaking screening instruments and that there may be cultural sensibilities around asking about psychological symptoms. There may also be a lack of effective interventions. Non-English speakers in the study were the least likely to be identified with mental health problems.

## DEPRESSION

Depression in pregnancy is significant. Gavin[4] et al in a review of depression in pregnancy and the postnatal period found that major depression was around 3.8% at the end of the first trimester, 4.9% at the end of the second and 3.1% at the end of the third. Postnatally it was highest at two months when it was 5.7% and 5.6% at six months.

Another study, Evans[5] et al, using self-reported measures, found higher rates at 32 weeks (13.5%) and eight weeks postnatally. Figures from NICE show a rate of 12% of women reporting symptoms of depression during pregnancy. Generally, it is considered that 1 in 5 women in the UK develop some mental health problems in pregnancy or in the following year, the most common being depression and/or anxiety. The direct effects of loss on this are difficult to measure and there is a lack of good research in this area.

An international literature review by Norhayati[6] et al into the magnitude and risk factors of postpartum symptoms, found on a self-reported questionnaire that the prevalence of postpartum depression varies between 1.9% and 82.1% in developing countries and from 5.2% to 74% in developed countries. There are considerable differences ranging from 0.1% in Finland to 26.3% in India. There are some concerns in using self-reporting but overall it gives some indications of women's state of mind. These figures are not differentiating those who have experienced loss from the general population of postpartum women.

Most health professionals are aware of postnatal depression and psychosis but may feel they are rare occurrences. They are much more likely to meet women with mild/moderate depression and generalised anxiety. A survey in published in 2017 by the RCOG and MMHA (Maternal Mental Health Alliance)[7] found that of 2,300 women surveyed who had given birth in the last five years 81% had experienced a mental health problem. Of these, over two-thirds reported low mood, half reported anxiety and a third depression. Only 7% of these women were referred for psychological support. Many experienced long waits for professional help and received little support for partners. Women waited anything from four weeks to a year and care varied enormously across the UK.

Depression is a common disorder, but it can be a disabling one and can affect not only the sufferer but also those around them. It is not just feeling low or sad. Everyone can feel that at times. It may bring feelings of hopelessness, anxiety, negativity and helplessness. The sense of loss of feelings of pleasure, low energy, poor concentration, and feelings of low self-worth, may not be recognised as symptoms of depression either by the sufferer or those around them.

Everyone's depression is individual but some of the symptoms are: loss of energy, sadness that persists, loss of self-esteem, feeling anxious all the time, and feeling helpless or hopeless. Sufferers may also feel guilt, have difficulty sleeping, loss of appetite and loss of libido. In more serious depressive episodes, they may also have thoughts of suicide or even make plans for it. Generally, it is characterised as MILD, with lack of concentration, low mood or lack of motivation, MODERATE where the above symptoms are more likely to interfere with day-to-day life and it may be deemed MAJOR, *i.e.* to need some therapeutic intervention, when daily life becomes very difficult and they may be at risk of harm. Whilst these categories are not exclusive, they may help the client to understand their illness. Bipolar Disorder also causes low mood as the sufferer will swing between high and low moods, although some may experience more of one than the other.

## TREATMENT OF DEPRESSION

Talking therapies have been shown to work well in depressive episodes. The type of therapy may depend on the preference of the client or on what is available, Cognitive Behaviour Therapy (CBT) and counselling are both helpful. CBT is a short-term structured therapy that helps to identify difficult areas and ways of thinking that are not helpful, and to look at how that may be changed. Counselling is less structured and can be open-ended, helping the client to explore past experiences and their effect on now and to look at how they can develop new strategies for coping. We will outline access to therapy in a later chapter. There is evidence for the value of CBT in postnatal depression and NICE recommends psychological therapies as a first line treatment for PND. In more severe depression, medication may be indicated. There are anti-depressants that can be taken during pregnancy. There are clear NICE guidelines available for the drugs that can be used safely in pregnancy and when breastfeeding.

A study by Wisner[8] *et al* reported that some depression following childbirth, especially among those considered more vulnerable, was helped by brief interventions included in the existing systems of help such as Planned Parenthood groups, antenatal classes and postnatal support groups.

> *Ellie was referred to the counsellor by her obstetrician when she recognised how low her mood seemed to be. She found it hard to discuss this with the midwives but was eventually persuaded to tell her story. Ellie lost her first son Joshua at seven weeks old. He had been delivered at 30 weeks with a heart disorder. He went into intensive care immediately after birth and had seemed to be doing well until six weeks when he started to go down. He died in intensive care and Ellie and her partner were distraught. She reported that all the staff in the unit were in tears and wanted to help but she just wanted to get away from the hospital and its connections.*

> *Ellie went back to work after a month, saying she "just tried to lose myself in work and not think". Her partner had packed away all the baby equipment and told family and friends, many*

*of whom lived overseas so were not available to support them. Ellie wanted to be pregnant again quickly and, after three months, she was. However, she did not expect to feel so low and tearful. She thought she would be joyful as she had been with Joshua. Her GP was concerned and thought she should see the Obstetrician as soon as possible. At this first meeting the doctor was happy with Ellie's physical health but very worried about her state of mind. She was exhibiting all the symptoms of depression. At the first appointment the therapist was also concerned, referring Ellie to a psychiatrist and making arrangements for regular therapy sessions. The psychiatrist wanted to prescribe antidepressants as she too felt the situation required treatment.*

*Ellie was concerned about taking the medication but the doctor convinced her that it was safe in pregnancy and she would be monitored throughout. Ellie admitted to the therapist that she had checked out the psychiatrist and the medication and was reluctantly agreeing to take it.*

*In the therapy sessions she was able to talk about the loss of Joshua and her feelings of failure. She felt that she had never failed at anything before and this should have been so easy. The sessions centred around this guilt and anger. Ellie did not think she would feel better until this baby was delivered, was well and reached eight weeks.*

*She continued taking the medication, having decided that this would be helpful for her and the baby. Ellie stayed on the antidepressants for three months and three months gradually reducing. By the time Rebecca was born she was still very anxious but not so low in mood. Therapy continued until Rebecca was two months old and Ellie was beginning to enjoy her. She was concerned that this meant that she had forgotten Joshua and needed to recognise that this was a normal reaction and that he would always be a part of her life.*

# OBSESSIVE-COMPULSIVE DISORDER (OCD)

OCD has two parts: obsession and compulsion. Obsessions are unwelcome and intrusive thoughts, images, worries or doubts that crop up repeatedly. They make the sufferer feel anxious or uncomfortable. These are often accompanied by the compulsions: repetitive activities such as checking an object maybe a door lock or kettle or how your body feels or repeating a phrase in your head. These activities feel out of control and may be frightening and unsettling.

Treatment is usually with medication and some talking therapies. Antidepressants are recommended by NICE and sometimes beta-blockers are given for the anxiety. Cognitive Behaviour Therapy has also been found to be effective. These treatments can be accessed via the GP although there may be waiting lists for therapy or specialist help.

A 2013 study of OCD by Russell[9] et a reported an increased rate of 1.5 to 2% in pregnant and postnatal women. It does not suggest the length of time the symptoms were experienced.

## ANXIETY OR GENERALISED ANXIETY DISORDER (GAD)

We cannot always separate anxiety from depression in the expressed feelings of the women or in the figures available. However, in a large US study Vesga-Lopez[10] et al found that 14.6% of mothers scored above the threshold in their rating scale at 18 weeks and 8% postnatally. Anxiety seems to increase postnatally, with panic disorders in particular worsening. Anxiety is a feeling of unease, worry and or fear that can vary from mild to severe. It is more than the normal feelings that everyone experiences in relation to an event or experience. When people have GAD, they cannot control their worries or fears. The anxiety is constant, and it affects their daily lives. They may experience physical symptoms such as shortness of breath or palpitations, feel restless and have trouble concentrating. Dizziness, dry mouth or excessive sweating may be experienced. Some may have panic attacks which can be very frightening. Some people are aware of their anxiety triggers and exploring this may help them to control the symptoms.

> Dina was delighted to be pregnant but was aware that she had experienced anxiety symptoms since her teens when she first left home. She went to university in her native Greece and moved to England with her partner five years ago. She had miscarried at eight weeks, soon after their arrival. She felt that she had been sad but coped well with the loss. She was now working in retail, which she enjoyed. As her pregnancy progressed, she began to feel anxious much of the time. She had not told her partner as she did not want to worry him. She felt a long way away from her parents in Greece who had been supportive in the past.

*Dina started to take time off work, blaming the pregnancy but actually because she became very anxious leaving the house and was reluctant to socialise. The midwife at her first appointment was able to help Dina to explain what was worrying her and referred her to the counsellor. Dina had experienced counselling before and understood the process but was afraid there would be questions about her ability to mother her child and was reluctant to re-engage with counselling.*

*By 30 weeks Dina was feeling unable to leave the house, was unable to manage her anxiety and her partner recognised what was happening. She agreed to see the GP, who was willing to prescribe for her but she refused, fearing it would harm the baby. Two weeks before her due date, she agreed to speak to the counsellor by telephone and was persuaded to come into the hospital, to speak to the counsellor and also to see the midwife, whom she had not seen since her first appointment. Dina agreed to come to a second appointment and to consider medication after her delivery. Dina and the counsellor agreed they would both speak to the GP after her delivery and that regular counselling sessions would be organised.*

## POST-TRAUMATIC STRESS DISORDER (PTSD)

Post-Traumatic Stress Disorder also showed an increased rate over the normal population immediately after a live birth, decreasing over the postnatal period, from 2.8% six weeks postnatally to 1.5% after six months. A paper by Susan Ayers[11] et al found that about a third of women in the western world evaluate their experience of childbirth as traumatic. 10% show some symptoms of trauma in the weeks following birth and 1-2% go on to develop PTSD that requires treatment. This would suggest that around 13,000 cases of postnatal PTSD arise every year in the UK alone. More recent work by Yildiz, Ayers and Phillips[12] suggests that 3%- 4% that is up to 28,000 UK women could be affected by maternal PTSD each year.

PTSD is a reaction to a traumatic experience. Trauma is the Latin word for wound, and people who are traumatised often feel wounded in body, mind and spirit. It may follow a sudden unexpected loss, a serious accident, seeing someone die, violence against oneself or someone close and experiences of war or terrorism. The illness means sufferers relive the event, which causes distress and disruption to their everyday life. The symptoms are similar to GAD: anxiety, hypervigilance and intense physical reactions to reminders of the event such as loud noises or memories triggered by pictures or conversations. These can cause the physical effects of anxiety such as pounding heart, nausea, tension and sweating, anger and fear.

A small study by Dr Jessica Farren[13] in the UK found that of her fairly small cohort, 28% met criteria for probable moderate to severe PTSD at one month after an early pregnancy loss (assessed on the Post -Traumatic Diagnostic Scale). 32% met criteria for moderate to severe anxiety and 16% for depression. At three months, the figures were 38% for PTSD, 20% for anxiety and 5% for depression. In the control group of those not experiencing pregnancy loss, none met the criteria for PTSD and 10% for depression and anxiety. The most commonly endorsed response on the questionnaire at one month was "feeling emotionally upset when reminded of the loss of your pregnancy". They also reported "upsetting thoughts or images of the loss which just came into your head" several times each week.

*Louise was slowly recovering physically after a very difficult forceps delivery. She visited her GP at six weeks and told her that she was experiencing flashbacks to the delivery which caused her to break out in sweats. She was also having panic attacks. Soon after she had gone home, she was anxious but thought this was normal and would go away as she settled into motherhood. Instead her symptoms had worsened and now her husband Des was concerned about her mental health. Her GP suggested starting anti-depressants but Louise was reluctant to take medication. The GP set up a counselling referral for Louise with the hospital and meanwhile suggested she looked on the MIND website for some support.*

*In the counselling sessions, as Louise took the counsellor through her experience, she began to recognise there were many things that had been lost through her childbirth journey. Louise had wanted to have a very natural birth. After all, many women seemed to give birth very easily and she had done all her preparation, including classes and yoga to get herself in the best possible situation for her labour. Des had been very involved with this and they had both looked forward to greeting their son.*

*In exploring the vast difference between her expectations and the reality, Louise began to recognise how badly and how much her beliefs had been shattered, how this had affected her and why she was feeling helpless and unable to make herself better. The details of her delivery had huge gaps which was also distressing her. The counsellor suggested she contacted the obstetrician to ask for an appointment to talk through what had happened in her labour and together they formed some of the questions that had been in Louise's mind. The appointment went well, and Louise did feel somewhat comforted to have some pieces of her jigsaw put into place.*

*When Louise could recognise that her labour had not gone badly because of something she had done then her thinking about the labour could change and slowly she was able to put the experience in a different place and concentrate on enjoying her beautiful, healthy son. Counselling had given her the opportunity to rethink and reframe a different way to look back at what had happened. There were missed opportunities in the early postnatal period. The possibility of developing some symptoms of PTSD could have been explained before the symptoms arose and signposts to information and support given to alleviate symptoms early.*

## TREATMENT FOR GAD AND PTSD

Talking therapies such as cognitive behaviour therapy are effective in treating GAD. A study by Otto, Smits and Reese, published by the American Psychological Association[14] found evidence for CBT as an effective treatment for anxiety disorders and offered maintenance of treatment gains, helping people to understand their symptoms and the causes of the anxiety. Therapy will also offer techniques to help to control or manage the feelings. Medication may help to relieve the symptoms and to help the client to feel more in control. There are self-help groups and online support available. Some of the value of these is not just the anonymity but also that they are available at any time. Anxiety does not wait for the next appointment. We will deal with these issues more fully in another chapter.

There is research, such as that by F Walsh[15], on not just treating PTSD as a mental illness with regular treatments, but also trying to develop resilience, as a way of helping individuals and families to feel more in control. For some people the symptoms of PTSD will gradually reduce over time, but for those in whom they persist, there is treatment available. This may be medication, CBT or both; or Eye Movement Desensitisation Reprocessing (EMDR). EMDR has been successful in treating PTSD reducing the negative thoughts and memories about a traumatic event. It involves the therapist usually moving a finger in front of the client as they follow side-to-side eye movements whilst recalling the traumatic event. It is thought that this replicates REM sleep, which in our everyday lives helps us to process emotional events. There do not seem to be any adverse effects of EMDR, although potential clients should be screened for suitability by the therapist. A review of the use of EMDR in other mental health conditions was published by A Valiente-Gómez[16] et al.

# EATING DISORDERS

Eating disorders are complex in their aetiology and treatment. They include any disordered eating patterns, starving, bingeing, purging and fasting. It is not only about the food or the body shape but also about control or coping mechanisms. The eating patterns may not be discreet but change and overlap. They are serious illnesses and untreated can lead to death. The stereotype of a young woman being the main sufferers may not be accurate as there is likely to be an undisclosed number among men and boys who do not present for help. The therapy is initially concerned with re-establishing healthy eating patterns. Some people are helped by talking therapies or self-help groups. However, once the weight loss or physical damage from bulimia is established, the client will need professional help. Treatment of eating disorders may need to be as an inpatient, although there are waiting lists and a limited number of beds in some areas.

Anorexia Nervosa is less common in pregnant women than in the general population because of reduced fertility as a result of the illness. Most women with bulimia nervosa have menstrual irregularities. However anorexic and bulimic women do become pregnant. Easter[17] et al suggest that 5-7.5% of pregnant women meet the criteria for an eating disorder. Watson[18] et al found preliminary evidence that pregnancy can lead to remission from bulimia but an increase in binge eating disorder. Women who have experienced eating disorders may be adversely affected by the changes in their body shape and size and by the feeling of this being out of their control.

A less common eating disorder but one sometimes related to pregnancy is Pica: the eating of items that are not food and have no nutritional value, such as soap, sponges, paint flakes, chalk or hair. There are no tests for diagnosis of Pica, but observation of the condition requires tests for anaemia or the toxic effects of some objects. It sometimes occurs with other mental health problems, but also in pregnancy, when it is thought to be related to iron deficiency anaemia or malnutrition, when treatment with vitamins may resolve it. The National Eating Disorder Association recommends that those who crave non-food items in pregnancy should only be diagnosed with Pica when their cravings pose a medical risk and they should be medically assessed. If mineral deficiencies have been checked and are normal, if the client and baby are considered to be at risk or the client is anxious or concerned, they can be referred for behavioural therapy. This may involve strategies for directing attention away from the items or a reward system for avoiding them.

There seems to be little research globally into eating disorders in pregnancy or the postnatal period. A small research study by Troop[19] et al exploring the social factors in the development of eating disorders found that women who developed an eating disorder were more likely to feel helpless in response to a crisis. This is significant in considering the effects of loss. They also reported that the onset of the symptoms of anorexia was associated with cognitive avoidance in a crisis, whilst those with bulimic symptoms were associated with cognitive rumination. Although a study in Norway by Watson[20] et al and reported in a meta-analysis, suggested that "some clinical studies found that women with a history of eating disorders, have a negative effect on birth outcomes".

> *Fay had been treated for anorexia as an in-patient in her mid-teens. Now 26 years old she was no longer anorexic but slightly underweight, very cautious about what she ate, and she still had times when she would start to weigh or measure her food. She was pregnant by choice by her boyfriend of three years.*
>
> *At her first appointment with the midwife, she brought a letter from her GP expressing some concern about her history of controlling her weight. She herself expressed some anxiety about managing her eating during her pregnancy, whether she needed to eat more than usual and what foods she should have. The midwife discussed this with her, and Fay said she thought she could manage it with her boyfriend's help. They considered talking to a dietitian but Fay was reluctant to revisit interactions from the past. As her body changed shape and she felt her weight increasing Fay expressed considerable anxiety and was referred to a Mental Health midwife for assessment and support. It helped Fay to feel that she had as much information and control as possible over the pregnancy and delivery. She became very anxious about a vaginal delivery and it was agreed that she would have a caesarean. Fay was followed up immediately after delivery by the mental health midwife she knew, and her care was transferred to the community mental health team.*

# PSYCHOSIS

Psychosis is a mental health disorder that causes people to experience hallucinations or delusions. Schizophrenia is the most common psychotic condition. Bipolar disorder, where mood can be low and then elevated, can also cause disturbing thoughts and behaviours in a "high" or manic state. Those who are suffering perceive or interpret things differently from those around them. They may have a lack of insight and self-awareness, with confused or disturbed thoughts.

Hallucinations are when someone sees or hears, smells, tastes or feels things that are not there. They may hear voices telling them to do things. Delusions are when people have an, often unshakeable, belief in something that is not shared by others. They may feel that people want to harm them or there is a conspiracy against them. Some may have grandiose ideas, where they believe they are someone with power or authority.

These ideas cannot usually be affected by talking to the client, or reasoning with them particularly as they may well not want to share their thoughts as part of the delusion. Medication is indicated as soon as the illness is recognised, as early treatment is often more effective. Talking therapies can offer support, particularly family intervention, which may reduce the need for hospitalisation. People with psychoses have a higher risk of self-harm and suicide, and of self-medicating with drugs or alcohol. Psychotic episodes can be frightening for the sufferer but also for those around them, who will need support to understand the course of the illness and its treatment.

*It was Beverley's first experience of working with postnatal women since qualifying as a midwife. She was enjoying working with their transition to motherhood and helping with establishing breastfeeding. One of the women she had been allocated was Rega who had given birth 3 days earlier to her daughter Freya. Rega was reported to be a little anxious and needing a lot of help with feeding her baby. At the start of her 12-hour shift, Beverley met Rega in her room and asked how her night had gone. Rega looked tired and anxious. Her night had been bad. She had had little sleep and angrily said, "This baby won't let me sleep. She is so demanding". In itself, this was not an unusual statement to hear from a first-time mother, so Beverley commiserated with her and said she would be back soon to examine both of them. 30 minutes later, Rega rang her bell. When Beverley went to her, Rega asked why she was back again so quickly. She seemed not to know she had rung her bell.*

*At the next breastfeeding session, both Beverley and Rega's mother were there. They both thought they were helping her with advice but Rega became quite angry with them for telling her different things and her anger only escalated when her partner arrived. By now, Rega was shouting loudly at everyone she saw and would not let go of Freya or put her down in her cot. Beverley became quits anxious about the safety of Freya and Rega. She asked a senior staff member to support her and to get a doctor review as a matter of urgency. By the time the medical staff arrived, the situation had escalated again and Rega was threatening to throw herself out of the window so everyone would stop shouting at her and her mother and partner were looking very frightened. The psychiatry team were called for and arrived to handle this escalating situation which was diagnosed as a psychotic episode.*

*Beverley had been very shocked at the rapidity of the developing symptoms with no warning. Rega had become very loud, accusing her of interfering and telling her and any other staff to get out of the room. It had left all the staff on shift quite shaken but they were comforted by the presence of one-to-one 24-hour care, which was delivered by the psychiatric staff who took some control over medication and supervision for the next few days.*

*Beverley came to talk through her worries at the end of the shift about the care she had given to Rega with the Specialist Midwife for Mental Health. She felt she may have been to blame for the situation becoming worse as she had been asking Rega questions. Beverley had missed the only session they had in their training that talked about mental health in childbearing so was totally unprepared as she had not experienced any situation like that before.*

*The specialist midwife suggested some simple steps to help during an episode, listen to the woman, tell her that she is acting differently and ask her to describe what she is experiencing. If appropriate, also tell her that what she is seeing or hearing is not real.*

*They talked through the background to psychosis and discussed some ideas about further information and research to look up.*

*Beverley said she would come back if she had any further concerns and wanted to continue caring for Rega and Freya.*

## TREATMENT OF PSYCHOSIS

In some areas and countries there are specialised perinatal mental health services. NHS England published a document in 2016 entitled Specialised Perinatal Mental Health Services (in-patient mother and Baby Units and Linked Outreach Teams) which covers mental health problems during pregnancy and up to one year after birth. It is a service specification for review by commissioning bodies in England. It was last updated in 2017 but at present there is no NICE Guideline. The Global Alliance for Maternal Mental Health campaigns for improved access and delivery of services for all women across the world with the backing of the WHO. `globalalliancematernalmentalhealth.org`

Women being treated for psychotic disorders were thought to be less fertile than the general population Howard[21] *et al* but changes in medication have led to less subfertility, particularly in bipolar disorder. The diagnosis of depression in pregnancy may mask an underlying bipolar disorder. Lydsdottir[22] found rates of 13% for Bipolar 2 in women with high levels of depressive symptoms in pregnancy and 22% postnatally. Prospective studies suggest an increased rate of relapse in pregnancy for women with bipolar disorder, particularly in the postnatal period. There does not seem to be any indication of the same course for schizophrenia during pregnancy. Postnatal psychosis characterised by both high and low mood, with a rapid onset and deterioration, including mood swings, delusions and/or hallucinations, generally occurs within two weeks after giving birth, but often in the first few days. Those with a previous history of bipolar disorder or postpartum psychosis are at high risk according to Robertson[23] *et al*. However, many women who experience a postpartum psychotic episode have no known history indicating high risk, as highlighted by Valdimarsdottir[24] *et al*. There is some evidence that complicated grief, that is when acute grief becomes debilitating, can increase the risk of mental ill health and needs some intervention.

## DRUG AND ALCOHOL MISUSE

Drug and alcohol use are common in the general population and therefore will be part of the life of some pregnant women. Drug misuse varies internationally in the drugs misused and the frequency of use. There are no national estimates in the UK for pregnant women who misuse drugs. Sherwood[25] *et al* and Williamson[26] *et al* in a study of inner-city maternity services drug screens, found 10%-15% of women using drugs, mostly cannabis although poly drug use was common. A US study in 1991 by Glantz and Woods[27] found up to 25% of pregnant women using illicit drugs. A 2015 study in the US by Forray[28] et al looked at the abstinence rates in pregnancy and the relapse rates postpartum over a two-year period. In their study, 83% of women achieved abstinence in at least one substance, cocaine, marijuana, cigarettes or alcohol. However, postpartum, 80% of women relapsed at least one substance. Women with a history of drug use are at the highest risk of relapse postpartum. Pregnancy abstinence rates were high for all substances except cigarettes. Postpartum 80% of women relapsed at least one drug most likely cigarettes and least likely cocaine. It may be that women substituted smoking for other drug use, and cigarettes are easily available and cheaper than most other drugs.

Substances of abuse fall into four main categories: stimulants such as cocaine and amphetamines; CNS depressants alcohol, sedatives, anxiolytics and hypnotics; opiates; and hallucinogens such as LSD and PCP. These are all associated with dependency. Women who have become dependent on drugs present complex physical and mental health problems. They have been found to smoke more, have poorer diets and low incomes They have a higher rate of maternal death and many received little healthcare. All these factors have an effect on foetal health and children's wellbeing. Many women do stop their drug use when they know they are pregnant but there is a high relapse rate, particularly if they do not have access to support and/or treatment.

> *Kate became pregnant whilst dependent on methadone. She lived a fairly chaotic lifestyle, moving from place to place and dependent for drugs, money and accommodation on her partner and on begging. Her partner, also an addict, was able to work and he received drugs from a clinic. She had not planned to be pregnant and did not attend any health facility until her partner took her with him to his Drug Dependency Clinic when she thought she was 24 weeks. The staff there talked to her to try to understand what she wanted to do and to persuade her to accept medical help. She was prepared to talk to them as she felt they were supportive of her partner, but that anywhere else would be critical and take the baby away. She was beginning to want to keep the baby but saw that she needed to make some changes, which frightened her. She agreed to go to an antenatal appointment if accompanied by the nurse practitioner from the drug clinic. She found the questioning, even about her health, quite intrusive and became aggressively defensive. She was persuaded to go on with it for the sake of the baby. With Kate's*

*permission, the clinic nurse talked to the midwife. They agreed that she would always see the same person and that the clinic would deal with her withdrawal from drugs. Kate did not find it easy to trust anyone. Having had an abusive childhood, she did not feel that anyone would care for her, but regular sessions with an understanding and non-judgmental midwife meant that she felt safer and could be persuaded that the baby would benefit. She tried to keep all interactions just about the baby. She was becoming increasingly concerned about losing the baby because of her previous behaviour. This fear of loss became her main focus. The midwife was aware that any questioning on her future plans made Kate angrily defensive and she would miss the next appointment. It was not possible for her to talk about this with Kate and the midwife recognised that she would have to work in a different way to support Kate and her baby, involving the few people that Kate felt she could trust.*

## ALCOHOL MISUSE

Alcohol use is common in the whole population. It is legal and easily available, so many pregnant women will have been drinking alcohol before they were pregnant and possibly early in the pregnancy, before it was confirmed. NHS guidelines and the Royal College of Obstetricians, as well as the RCM, recommend that pregnant women do not drink alcohol at all during their pregnancy and if they are breastfeeding. The dangers for those with low to moderate consumption are a slightly increased risk of having a baby small for dates. A study by the University of Bristol[29] found an 8% increased risk of a baby small for dates in women who had low to moderate alcohol consumption. Although this meta-analysis found no significant difference in the average birth weight between drinkers and non-drinkers across seven studies, they reported that overall there was insufficient research in this area to draw definitive conclusions and that there is "limited evidence for a causal role of light drinking in pregnancy compared with abstaining on most of the outcomes examined."

Heavy drinking has been found to cause early miscarriage, premature birth and Foetal Alcohol Syndrome. A study by the Canadian Institute for Mental Health Policy Research found that Britain came seventh out of 195 countries for the proportion of children with Foetal Alcohol Syndrome (FAS)[30]. The researchers looked at 24 global studies and found that 32 in 1000 Britons have FAS, 15 in 1000 in the US and 10 in France. FAS can have serious effects on the child, including poor growth and severe mental and developmental problems.

The loss of the perfect baby for these women is of serious concern and they may need to recognise the extent of their drinking and the damage it may cause and find help to stop drinking. There may be some difficult conversations for the midwife around the amount someone is drinking and the effect on the foetus. Women may not understand the effects of alcohol and may then feel guilty about her drinking. This may result in distress or a defensive reaction. For women who cannot or will not stop drinking, the midwife can discuss the risks with them and perhaps refer them to a mental health specialist or they can be signposted to Alcoholics Anonymous (AA) or Drinkline, a national telephone support agency. Being given some idea of what to expect if they contact one of these organisations may help them to feel more positive about it.

## HEALTH PROFESSIONALS AND THE CARE OF PATIENTS WITH MENTAL HEALTH ISSUES

The NHS Mandate sets the objective to "reduce the incidence and impact of postnatal depression through early diagnosis and better intervention and support". However, the Royal College of Obstetricians and Gynaecologists and Maternal Mental Health report 2017 states that, "women frequently reported that they received inconsistent and conflicting advice around medication and those who voiced concerns were shut down or had to repeatedly ask for help." This is clearly an area that needs to be addressed by those seeing women early in the pregnancy but who may feel they do not have sufficient expertise in this area. Encouraging the woman to talk to her GP or psychiatrist and showing her that she will be supported in this may allow her to feel safe. For many of these women suffering from anxiety and low mood, it may be that being gently reminded they have a space in which they can express their feelings and fears and will be heard may be enough to hold them until they receive professional mental health care. Indeed, some may find that is enough in itself.

The report continues:

> *"Healthcare professionals are often the first point of contact that a woman suffering with mental health problems reaches out to and we must ensure that all staff involved in the care of women during pregnancy and the first year after birth have relevant education and training in perinatal mental health. Our role should increasingly be about empowering women to make*

*decisions about their care and in supporting women to help themselves."*

A report in the Nursing Times in 2007 of a survey by the PANDAS Foundation and the Community Practitioners and Health Visitors Association indicated a lack of training and knowledge of mental health in pregnancy. 72% of midwives and health visitors in the survey said that they did not think the amount of training on pre and postnatal mental illness was enough. 39% did not feel they had the appropriate skills and knowledge to deal with a patient who presented with a prenatal mental illness from diagnosis to referral and follow-up.

Some health professionals do not feel equipped by training or experience to deal with mental health issues when they are presented as such, but it may be that by asking relevant questions and using some basic counselling skills that can be adapted to the situation and the time available. These staff members can offer invaluable support and help. To identify depression and/or anxiety, you can ask, "Have you recently, perhaps in the last month, felt down, depressed or hopeless? Have you felt less pleasure in doing things that you would have enjoyed in the past?" For concern about anxiety, "Have you felt nervous, on edge or anxious?" and "Have you found it hard to stop worrying?". If the answers are positive in a way that seems much more than usual for the woman, it is possible to use Depression Identification Scales or to refer the woman for counselling, if she is willing and if it is available to her GP. It is also important to the health professionals and the woman and her family to feel confident in enquiring at booking about her previous mental health and any treatment she has received.

This may indicate a need for medication assessment during pregnancy, or just an awareness that she may be at risk. In many hospitals, there are obstetricians and specialist midwives working as a team with women with mental health issues. They will be able to advise other members of the healthcare team. There is very clear information available on the suitability of psychotropic drugs in pregnancy.

Many of the concerns expressed by women in the RCOG mental health survey were around the lack of continuity of care and the experience of care being rushed and impersonal. The women questioned were not so concerned about the job title of the person they were talking to, but how comfortable they felt. They found it hard to confide in someone they may not see again. It may be that this is inevitable and so the professional who does have the time or access to the patient needs to make the most of that opportunity. Many women found that there was not a time when they felt comfortable to disclose their feelings. Those who did, found it helpful and it was often all they needed at that time. Many expressed concerns about the information being on their medical records. The RCOG report found that this was the biggest reason for not wanting to disclose any mental health issues. This information may need to be recorded and the value of this can be explained to the client.

NICE recommends that every woman be asked about her emotional wellbeing at first, and every subsequent, contact with health professionals. These should include questions about her mood and her personal circumstances, including domestic violence and drug and alcohol use. The two central questions about mental health, known as the Whooley Questions are: "During the past month, have you often been bothered by feeling down, depressed or hopeless?" and "During the last month have you often been bothered by little interest or pleasure in daily things". The Whooley questions were found to elicit a disorder as well as the longer Edinburgh Postnatal Depression Scale (Howard 2018). The study in the British Journal of Psychiatry concluded that:

*"The endorsement of the Whooley questions indicates the need for a clinical assessment of diagnosis and could be implemented when maternity professionals have been appropriately trained on how to ask the questions sensitively, in a setting where a clear referral and care pathway is available."*

The RCOG report found that 52% had been asked about their emotional health by a midwife, 67% by a health visitor, 31% by a GP and 4% by an obstetrician.

This leaves a large group who were never asked about their feelings, even before the very low numbers of referrals. Women with a history of mental illness were more likely to be referred to a mental health practitioner. Of those not referred, many sought help outside NHS services. Some turned to family or friends, 28% sought help through online services and 12% found private counselling. A number were helped by charities and community groups, activity groups or mother and baby groups. All these are good sources of support and comfort but may not be enough for those women with an identifiable mental illness.

Specialist Mental Health Midwives are now working in the NHS offering a resource to clients and staff, with the identification of mental health problems and expertise on assessment, treatment availability, the teaching of other staff and mentoring for midwives. They are also working closely with specialist obstetricians and linking with the psychiatric team.

# THE MENTAL HEALTH OF THE PROFESSIONALS

Health professionals may, just as in the general population, have or have had their own mental health issues. Brooks[31] *et al*, in a review of literature on the mental health of doctors, found that mental ill health was common among doctors, who were often reluctant to seek help. They suggest there is a wealth of research indicating that doctors have high rates of mental health problems, including depression, anxiety and addiction to drugs and alcohol. Suicide levels are higher than in the general population, particularly for female doctors. The risk factors are considered to be occupational, structural, clinical and personal. These include the high expectations of themselves and others and the aggression they experience in some branches of medicine. The long, unsocial hours, the lack of teamwork and support, conflict with colleagues and bullying all contribute. Personal factors include perfectionism, unhelpful coping strategies, a desire to please and guilt for things beyond their control. Mark and Smith[32] found healthcare workers, and particularly nurses, to be among those who fall into the high stress category, with NHS nurses the most likely to experience high levels of stress. Whilst this in itself is not a mental disorder, it can lead to burnout and depression, absence from work and the possibility of affecting patient care.

Staff are often reluctant to seek help, feeling embarrassed, or that they are being weak or from fear of negative career effects. This is also reflected in a Canadian study by Moll[33] who found health care professionals have a high level of workplace stress and a higher risk of mental health problems than the general population. They tend not to seek help but experience tensions in the workplace, damage to their reputation and have the potential for compromising patient care. The study recommends the use of Mindfulness techniques. Several large studies in Canada and the USA quoted in the same review found that 15-20% of healthcare professionals would probably or definitely not seek help with emotional problems. Becoming a patient is a big hurdle for many health workers.

This qualitative analysis was consistent in showing that overall, mental health problems in the healthcare workplace were dealt with by silence and inaction. This arose from an uncertainty in identifying mental health issues and the stigma that was attached to them. Further, the concern about confidentiality and a lack of access to support. The difficulty of knowing where to seek help seems to be another reason for inaction.

The Royal College of Nurses 2005 Working Well Survey found that on a CORE questionnaire 40% of nurses showed signs of psychological ill health, 14% minimal, 12% moderate and 14% in distress. They found no discernible differences between men and women or in relation to ethnic origin. Nurses responding to the survey said that stress was reduced by employee friendly work patterns, the opportunity for training and development, supportive supervision and flexible working. Reduced stress was linked to job satisfaction.

A study by Jonas-Simpson[34] *et al* explored the grief nurses experienced after a perinatal death. This was a small in-depth study, which found that the grief they experienced the personal and professional impact was reduced by receiving and giving meaningful help; support from colleagues, education and mentoring. They required acknowledgement, support and education.

Whilst there are now more mental health literacy programmes, that wider knowledge does not always bring with it sympathetic attitudes. These need to come from supportive leadership and management as well as teams who understand and support colleagues without fear. Some areas have tried to offer support to staff with mental health issues offering confidential services outside the workplace. A study in the USA by Shapiro[35] using mindfulness techniques for stress reduction in health care staff found that an eight-week intervention may be effective for reducing stress, improving the quality of life and increasing self-care.

## ACCESS TO MENTAL HEALTH CARE

The provision of Mental Health Care in the UK is administered under the Mental Health Act 2007, which is the UK legislation covering the assessment, treatment and rights of people with a mental health disorder. It requires assessment by approved mental health clinicians. The Act provides criteria for compulsory admissions known as involuntary commitment, definitions of mental disorder and the provision of a Mental Health Tribunal, as well as details about particular treatments. Access to care in the UK is usually via a GP. The GP can refer to hospital psychiatric services, and they may also be able to access community support with therapists, mental health nurses and psychologists. There is an 18-week maximum waiting time. The difficulty is always the waiting time to access any service: 18 weeks may seem far too long to someone in distress. Those with the finances or with insurance may be able to go to private psychiatric hospitals or clinics.

Some services accept self-referral. These are mainly for drug and alcohol misuse. Services for young people are run by CAMHS (Child and Adolescent Mental Health Services). They will accept referrals from parents and teachers, as well as GPs.

There are no services specifically provided by the NHS for bereavement, although they may exist in some areas, often run by charities such as Cruse or local support groups. The NHS Choices website signposts local services.

Specialist care for postnatal depression and psychosis is not always available in a client's area. If they need to be admitted it may be to a mother and baby unit, which can be some distance away. Follow up will be by the community mental health team, but this of course requires a change of caring staff. Where there is no mother and baby bed available the mother may be admitted alone if she needs urgent care.

The NHS Choices website provides a guide to the services available and makes clear when you have a choice. There are signposts on the site which direct the user to support services and directories for different mental health conditions.

# THE EFFECTS OF LOSS ON THE PROFESSIONALS

Anyone helping and supporting someone who experiences a loss cannot avoid being affected by it. We are people first, before we are professionals. Our own experiences and culture will impact on how we regard loss and mourning. Some may react immediately, crying with the family or the woman, or they may carry out their professional tasks at the time and react later. There is a conflict around what is appropriate professional behaviour and having a personal response to a difficult experience. How people respond depends in part on their level of attachment to the bereaved, on their own coping strategies, and the availability of support. There are many ways to cope with such an experience: some helpful, some less so. For some people, denial is the way they cope at the time. Some may withdraw from the family, which may make it difficult to deal with the needs of the client and their own needs. They do not acknowledge their feelings and get on with being 'professional'. This denial and withdrawal may be associated with feeling helpless or being unprepared to manage the feelings; or it may relate to unresolved grief of their own.

It is important that health professionals are aware of their own experiences of grief and how it may still be affecting them. Understanding this may help them to understand the grief of their clients without becoming part of it. Saunders and Valente[36] found that health professionals given advice and training on the theories of loss and grieving and the tasks of mourning, felt more able to develop their own helpful coping strategies. These may mean rationalising what has happened, reflecting on how it was managed and accepting the event. It is not possible to plan for these events and each one will be different, so protocols are of limited use.

It is being able to understand the needs of the client and how the health professional can offer support with warmth and genuineness, that will make everyone feel heard and cared for. Downey[37] et al found staff could recall the experiences of loss after a considerable period of time, with identifiable triggers in the workplace. Some also reported intrusive reflections in their domestic situation. Understanding that this can happen may help them to manage the fears and feelings.

Marris[38] suggests four kinds of conditions influencing an ability to cope with loss, both for clients and staff. They are: childhood experiences and the feelings of security engendered; conflict over the meaning of what is lost; sudden unexpected loss and relationships after loss, including how much support is available.

Support and empathy from colleagues are of real importance after a loss, particularly an unexpected or sudden one. It reduces the feelings of isolation and the questioning of guilt and responsibility. In a critical review of literature relating to midwives' and nurses' response to neonatal loss, Wallbank[39] et al they found that notable to all the accounts they reviewed was the "overarching theme of staff isolation "and the perception of limited or absence of organisational support and resources. A time to reflect without blame or guilt outside of official reviews can be hugely helpful. Some staff may feel that looking for or needing support affects their professional image of always being able to cope. Not only is it likely to benefit them it also enhances their professional image as someone who is open, empathetic and sensitive. Insensitive comments can impact greatly on staff as well as clients, as research published by Doka[40] demonstrates, and can affect their ability to cope with stressful situations in the future. Healthcare professionals may need to seek out this support and, in some cases, may need to look outside their workplace. Some may need to take time away from work or from direct client involvement if they recognise that they are finding it difficult to engage with clients. Where there are effective mentoring systems in place and particularly support for students and people early in their careers, it can help them to feel more confident to cope with these difficult situations and find their own ways to deal with them.

No one can teach someone how to deal with each difficult loss that occurs but coping strategies that work for you give you structure and a greater feeling of safety. We cannot eliminate risk and however 'risk management' is discussed and implemented, midwives and nurses deal with uncertainty all the time, and some situations cannot be controlled or managed. Then people are thrown on their own resources and the support that they are able to find. We sometimes talk about closure, by which we mean moving on from an event, but should also include resolution and acceptance. We may not be able to forget but we can accept the event happened and that we need to move forward. It helps to know we acted appropriately, and to the best of our abilities. No one gets it right all the time. Support from colleagues and being able to express their feelings help many staff to move forward and feel that they have learned from the experience. Some health professionals will be experiencing, or will have experienced, mental health problems of their own. Caring for the carers is an important part of training and practice.

# 6: Counselling Skills and Models of Counselling

*Counselling skills for health professionals; the basic skills of counselling; attending and listening; goal setting; empathy; warmth and genuineness; the don'ts; models of counselling.*

## COUNSELLING SKILLS FOR HEALTH PROFESSIONALS

Effective professional "helpers" are aware of both the physical and emotional needs of their clients but also aware of their own experiences and feelings. All helping is done within a relationship that requires input from both sides. This is not to say that a helper has to reveal themselves to a client but that they are aware of their own responses, their prejudices and needs. It is within this relationship of trust and respect that both client and helper will feel safe, and their well-being encouraged. Counselling or any kind of therapy is not about making people happy. It may never achieve that outcome, but it is about helping to find a way forward that fits the needs of the client and to accept and manage thoughts and feelings. It should then be suitable and available to all clients where there is no language difficulty. For those clients, it may be necessary to find a speaker of the same language or to use an interpreter.

Just by becoming 'a patient', people can feel that they regress to childhood when they needed help to care for themselves and advice and information. This may be comfortable for many and most know how to be a "good patient", but for others the lack of control may mean a loss of self and independence. It may also mean fear or apprehension about the unknown. Loss makes people experience feelings that they may never know in any other circumstances. The anger is greater, the distress can feel unbearable and life will never be quite the same again. People may feel shock or disbelief at some outcomes, particularly when they experience a loss. They can also feel guilt or shame that they have not managed to produce a live, healthy baby, or that they are not coping with their feelings.

This is when using counselling skills to help an individual, family or couple to move forward can provide a great deal of support and a way to see the future. In all their work, health professionals give advice, information, coaching or instruction. The skills that will help those who cannot see where they are or where to go are different. Counselling is the process of helping someone to see their way from the uncomfortable place they are in now to a future, safer and more comfortable place. There are various types of intervention. These may be informative, prescriptive or comforting. Most situations health professionals will recognise. They may also be challenging, cathartic and supportive.

## THE BASIC SKILLS OF COUNSELLING

There are some models of counselling that may be used for longer or short-term contact with clients but the skills of the helper are the same and can be used by everyone who interacts with people needing help or support. There are numerous books and courses at all levels for anyone wanting to explore and develop their skills.

There are also online courses that may give health professionals some confidence in using this approach. The skills that are universal to all the approaches are: attending and listening, goal exploring and goal setting and challenging the thoughts and feelings that keep clients stuck in a difficult place.

These skills are all part of how we can help people to move on and to develop their own strategies for coping. These are techniques that can be used by everyone and need only self-awareness and an opportunity to make a relationship, however brief, with the client. It requires an empathic relationship, that is an ability to enter their internal world, to see it in some way through their eyes, and to let them know that you are accepting their feelings.

The skills of the counsellor are listening, genuineness, warmth, insight and non-judgmental response. Many health professionals are doing some or all of these in their daily interactions but when the relationship is one of direct involvement in a person's feelings, there has to be more awareness of self in the relationship and what you are trying to achieve, allowing the client to feel free to express any feelings and have them taken seriously, considered and reflected. The concentration is always on the client's problems. These skills arise from an awareness of yourself, your own prejudices, responses and sensitive areas, and how you relate to people. They can be practised and developed. No one gets it right all the time but recognition of helpful interactions, reflection on what you say and how it is received all hone the skills and bring confidence in using them.

## ATTENDING AND LISTENING

Attending is truly focusing outwards on the client. We are allowing them the space to talk and the respect for what they are telling us. We have to be careful not to judge what they are saying or to be distracted by our own responses. Our reactions are part of the process but if we make assumptions without checking with the client, we are dealing with our own feelings and not theirs.

When we become conscious of really focusing, we also become aware of the times that this is difficult: when we are tired or distracted by a problem of our own, for example, then we cannot properly attend to the client. We may need to keep re-focusing during a session in order to stay in touch with the person in front of us.

Listening is about being able to hear the other person; not just what they are saying but all aspects of their communication. This may be the words they use to convey feelings, or the spaces between words and phrases, the tone or pitch of their voice. The metaphors they use, the way they describe things and their words, all give us insight into their internal world. Non-verbal communication, body position or movement, gestures, facial expressions and touch are all part of how we communicate. Someone who reaches out to touch the counsellor may need reassurance or to feel that they are being heard. We need to notice these things but not to make assumptions and to check with the client. "It seems like you are...." may give them permission to express their feelings.

## GOAL SETTING

In short-term counselling, or just in a supportive framework, it can help the client to set realistic goals. Breaking down a problem into small parts and planning strategies for dealing with those make it feel more manageable and also more rewarding when those goals are reached. For someone who has felt too anxious to leave the house, planning to go into the garden or meet a friend on the street may be a huge step but they may find they can manage this if they do not try to do too much; and to congratulate themselves when they achieve it. Giving and receiving feedback is an important part of this process.

## EMPATHY

Empathy is imagining how it would be to be the other person. It is not sympathy which is imagining I am the other person and how I would feel. Perhaps feeling sorry for them. When we empathise with someone, we do not know the outcome we take the journey alongside them, not thinking of answers or solutions, not judging or making suggestions. We may reflect back to the client what they are saying, often in their words, so that they can hear what they are saying and feeling.

## WARMTH AND GENUINENESS

This suggests an openness to the client, and an approachability, which is particularly important to those new to talking about their feelings or those who are in pain. It is treating the other person as a human being but not as a friend. In situations where you may be alongside parents who have lost a child, it is normal to express your feelings for them, to maybe touch them and recognise their pain, but the relationship is always about them. They are coming to you for help, and we cannot expect the warmth we express to be returned. Genuineness means being interested, fake concern is always spotted and there can be no trust in the relationship if it is felt to false. We cannot always be interested in a situation, but we can be committed to it.

## THE DON'TS

There are some "don'ts" in the counselling process, at whatever level we engage with it. Avoid interpretations - that is, do not offer an explanation of the person's thinking, feelings or behaviour. That can be helpful but is best done by the client. If I interpret what they are saying, it may be based on my feelings or experiences.

We all deal with things differently and have lived a different life, so our experience will affect how we think and behave and will not be the same as someone else's. If we ask open questions such as, "I wonder if ..." or, "What do you think/feel about ...", we will help the client to examine their own feelings and actions.

Advice can be unhelpful except when there are clear facts. Midwives, nurses and doctors sometimes find this difficult, as so much of their role is to offer clear advice and guidance. In the counselling situation it can make someone feel directed or judged. This may lead someone to go against their own judgement or they may feel dependent on the counsellor, or perhaps feel a failure when they are unable to take the advice. Avoid "oughts" and "shoulds". Most people want to please those who are trying to help. Giving advice or direction can mean that they do not think things through for themselves, or if they feel things go wrong, they may lose trust in the helper.

Try not to invalidate a client's feelings. In trying to make them feel better it is easy to say, "Oh, that's not right" or, "You shouldn't feel like that". We need to listen to what they are feeling and help them to see the rightness or wrongness of their feelings or behaviours for themselves. If we do not do this, it may seem like the counsellor is better placed to assess the client's feelings than they are themselves. It is always the clients' recognition of their feelings and behaviours that we are trying to help them reach.

# MODELS OF COUNSELLING

There are many models of counselling. Not all will be right for everyone as a practitioner as well as a consumer. The choice may be based on what is available as well as what will be most effective. It is also important that the client feels comfortable with the therapist or counsellor, as well as with the approach to therapy. Clients need to feel clear about what is being offered. This may be, "I can only see you for a few sessions," when it may be important to focus on certain goals.

Some therapy needs a longer commitment and again the client needs to understand what that may be, even if we are just referring someone on. It is important that people are referred to a qualified therapist in whichever form of therapy. This can be quite difficult to check but clients or potential clients need to ask what training and qualifications someone has. There are registers of counsellors and therapists, some of which are available online. These may not be vetted for qualifications. Recommendations and word of mouth may be a way to find a reputable therapist.

It is not the purpose of this book to give extensive information about therapies. This can be found on the internet or from the various organisations outlined at the end of the book. We have included some of the most commonly and reliably used approaches to therapy, to give people new to the area some ideas on what may be suitable and available.

## PSYCHODYNAMIC THERAPY OR PSYCHOANALYSIS

This is a longer-term therapy practised by qualified therapists and analysts, using the theories of Freud, Jung and Klein among others. It emphasises the effect of the past on the present, exploring a person's early life and childhood relationships with parents and family to consider how this has shaped their personality, ways of thinking and behaving, and their current relationships. The model accepts that much of what we experienced in childhood is still in our unconscious mind and influencing our present thoughts and behaviours. Psychodynamic therapy encourages the client to explore memories of significant events and feelings that help the client to understand the present. This work takes time and commitment and the training is quite long requiring an in-depth knowledge of the theories.

## COGNITIVE BEHAVIOUR THERAPY (CBT)

CBT is concerned with changing the way you think and behave. It is based on the concept that thoughts, feelings and actions are inter-connected and negative thoughts keep you in a negative place. This cycle of negativity can be, "I feel low/depressed" or, "I've let everyone down and I'm a bad friend", leading to social withdrawal; or, "I feel low/depressed and no-one will want to be with me". The therapy helps to break down the overwhelming feelings into small parts to explore the negative and unhelpful beliefs that can lead to a change in thinking and thus a change in feelings and behaviour. It aims to give people the tools to do this for themselves, when they recognise that they are thinking negatively. It has been used online and with distance/telephone support quite successfully. There are self-help books and internet-based programmes. CBT is used most commonly for anxiety and depression but may also help in other mental health conditions. It can be accessed via some GPs or private practitioners.

## CRISIS COUNSELLING

This is designed to offer swift, short-term help and support to help people regain effective functioning particularly after unexpected loss or illness. It aims to help a person to face up to the crisis and avoid denial. To break up the crisis into manageable parts so that people do not feel overwhelmed and can see things they can do to move forward. It requires the counsellor to avoid taking over and to help the client to use their own resources and develop or recognise their own coping mechanisms. False reassurance that, "Everything will be ok" will not sound genuine and will not help the client to find their own resources and strategies for coping. Often, people can be helped to see how they have coped in previous situations and to recognise that they do have helpful strategies once they do not feel overwhelmed. Helping to set realistic goals in the short term can free people from feeling that they have to "have everything sorted" at once and be able to cope with everything.

## MINDFULNESS

Mindfulness is about knowing what is happening inside and outside ourselves from moment to moment. Awareness of our environment, the sounds around us or the feeling of a chair or the breeze, and also our internal world of thoughts and feelings. Professor Mark Williams, former Director of the Oxford Mindfulness Centre, writes that, "it is easy to stop noticing the world around us, to lose touch with the way our bodies are feeling and to end up living in our heads, caught up in our thoughts without stopping to notice how those thoughts are driving our emotions and behaviour."

Becoming aware of the moment can help us to set aside some repetitive thoughts or brooding and to stand back and see the patterns of our thoughts and behaviours. It helps us to notice signs of stress and anxiety and to try to give ourselves space to allow our thoughts to clear.

Mindfulness is a kind of meditation that is improved by practice and regular use. Even five minutes as you travel to work or pack the lunch, gives you that space. You can start to be aware of how your immediate environment feels, the noises on the bus, the rain on the window or the smell of the bread as you make a sandwich. This gives time away from intrusive or troubling thoughts, and an awareness of how we are feeling in our bodies and our minds. It is not about making difficult thoughts or problems go away but seeing them as events that are part of ourselves. There is some evidence that Mindfulness can help with anxiety and depression and it is recommended by NICE. There are some online self-help courses, as well as private therapists and some counsellors in GP practices.

Yoga and Tai Chi can also help those who prefer a physical and meditational way of reaching a similar place. These are available locally and some are funded by local further education or supported by the NHS. Some people with depression especially find benefit in physical exercise. It can be anything that suits the person, whether alone or in a group. The endorphins help the psychological state, as does the feeling of doing something positive for yourself.

There are other therapies that are available and can be found on the internet or in some places via the GP or the local health service. Information about all the different types of therapy is available online and through the organisations that govern them. There are guides to what therapy involves and choosing a counsellor or psychotherapist published by the Counselling Directory and the UKCP the UK Council for Psychotherapy.

# 7: Communication

*Effective communication; communicating with partners; complex situations; training in communication; breaking bad news; complicated communication; managing anger; caring for the professionals; understanding cultural differences; private time with the baby; issues for staff; decision-making; social media.*

Communicating is what most of us do, most of the time. Communicating effectively, especially in a healthcare setting, is more challenging. It depends on making a quick and helpful relationship and giving information and support in a way that people can receive. Communicating information is vital in all aspects of healthcare and it needs to be communicated in a way that makes the client feel comfortable enough to engage with what is being said; and encourages feedback to enhance memory and check that the clients feel heard and are able to hear. Good communication, even in brief interchanges, improves client satisfaction and reduces anxiety.

Finding out what the client wants to know is the start of information giving. Then it is possible to relate the explanation to the expectations. This will help the client hear what is said and it will feel congruent with their feelings and needs. If information is given clearly and often when clients are in distress, in more than one form, they will have a chance to think or talk about it later. If you ask for feedback, it is helping the healthcare professional and the client to check understanding and recall.

People feel dissatisfied with communication when it does not meet their needs, this may be the context, the language or the timing of the interaction. Clients do not always feel able to ask questions and giving clear space for this can be helpful. The sense of healthcare professional and client working as a team encourages everyone to communicate better. Clients feel more engaged and able to ask questions and challenge expectations.

## EFFECTIVE COMMUNICATION IN HEALTHCARE

The literature in the last decades has delivered more emphasis on effective communication in healthcare practice. Simpson[1] *et al* found that good practice includes relationship building, taking patient's feelings into account and understanding the patient's perspective and including the client in decision-making. Stewart[2] and other studies have found that good communication in health care is associated with positive outcomes such as increased client satisfaction, the adjustment of expectations and better coping.

Communicating with clients with special needs may require external help. Health professionals may need to check with clients with hearing loss how they feel most comfortable communicating. Some will be used to lip reading others may need someone with them who can sign. There may be a loop system available. For those with vision problems, signposting them to helplines may make it easier for them to access information. This may have to be done through a companion. There are large print and braille blog tags available via NHS UK.

*Soo and her partner Sam had experienced a miscarriage at 15 weeks, two years before they came for a booking appointment for her second pregnancy. She was extremely anxious and her English, which was usually good, began to desert her when she became tearful. The midwife asked her about the loss and with Sam's help she described what had happened at home and then the admission to hospital. She did not understand why it had gone wrong and could not remember being told anything. Sam said that the doctor had given them no real explanation beyond, "These things happen ... you can try again"; and had ignored the fact that English was a second language for Soo.*

*Soo thought it might have been her fault that she could not understand the language that was used and that she was given no space to ask questions at a time when Sam was there to help her. Sam felt that they could have offered an interpreter to help Soo to understand the explanations. Soo felt that she must be responsible for the loss but could not think what she had done wrong and had gone over and over what she might have done.*

*The midwife carefully explained what would happen next and listened to what the couple were expecting. Soo still felt unable to ask anything and the midwife suggested she read a leaflet and try the internet which would give her time to think. The midwife also suggested that she would try to find out any further information about the miscarriage for them. Soo and Sam felt heard this time and that just having someone take time and care reduced some of the anxiety. They were able to ask what they could do that might prevent another miscarriage and whether they could talk to someone if Soo was anxious.*

# COMMUNICATING WITH PARTNERS

Pregnancies do not just belong to the woman carrying the baby and partners can be fully invested in each step along the way. Engaging with them and keeping them involved throughout the pregnancy loss experience is an important part of caring. Whilst women in most cultures have access to support from other women after the loss of a pregnancy or baby, men appear not to have the same support offered to help them through their feelings. Little research has been done to elicit the impact on men of the trauma of loss or difficult delivery or even loss of their partner. What research is available supports the theory that there are gender differences in responses, therefore their needs differ. This is vital to recognise to ensure they get the help they need through and after such a devastating event in their lives.

In a systematic review of the literature available on the impact of pregnancy loss on men's health and wellbeing in 2017 Men and Pregnancy Loss[3], Due et al sampled 29 articles, both qualitative and quantitative, from around the world. It was generally found that men did report many of the same feelings as women, but they were less intense and for a shorter period. Whilst men generally saw their role was as a supporter, they felt others did not identify that they were suffering too. That can be exacerbated by the fact that women have the physical aspects of loss to manage as well as the emotional whilst the men stand by and watch. This can be very disempowering, involving them in discussions about the range of emotions that may be felt by both partners can help them to be able to identify their feelings and give them permission to show them in all their rawness.

Men sometimes report that they do not always find it easy to access their emotions so may not be able to display their feelings. This may be a personal or a cultural effect on their experience. In a newspaper article in 2014 about the experience of a miscarriage Terry Maguire[4] said, "Her (his wife's) emotions were so raw and obvious that there was no mistaking what she was experiencing. While on the face of it I was just getting on with things and appeared very quickly to have put the upset behind me". He goes on to say this was far from the truth, but he kept his feelings hidden in an effort to be strong for her. This reminds us that the questions about feelings are a very important part of the care provided to couples and asking men and repeating over time, "How are you feeling?" may just give them the opportunity they need to disclose.

In some cultural situations, ventilation of feelings is not encouraged and men are left anxious about feeling vulnerable or weak. This is most definitely a time to acknowledge their loss, to listen to them, to quietly support them and allow them to express their feelings without judgement.

Men and women also may use returning to work after a loss as an avoidance mechanism in order to distract them from their feelings and in an effort to locate some control in a confusing situation. This does not always help and may only delay grief until a later time. Sometimes it cannot be avoided, and people may need help to manage this and to ask for support from employers.

Little is known about the effects on same-sex partners and how they cope with loss in their relationships. As pregnancies are now created in different ways and in many different relationships, there is a need for research into the effects of loss in non-heterosexual relationships and donor and surrogate pregnancies to help professionals improve the care they offer to all involved in the creation of these pregnancies. For now, the caregivers will need to be aware of the impact of loss on all the parties to the pregnancy.

## COMPLEX SITUATIONS

Some areas of care require particular communication skills. In assisted reproduction, where success rates are quite low and treatment is a huge source of stress for couples and individuals, good communication can be crucial to retention in care, shared decision making and the reduction of distress. Gameiro[5] et al and others have found that poor communication and relationships with clinic staff was a cause of dissatisfaction, and one of the reasons clients stopped treatment or changed clinics. They reported that discontinuation was due to communications being insufficient, poor explanations about fertility problems, poor management of psychological aspects and inadequate provision of information.

Huppelschoten[6] et al in Holland looked at the drop-out rate for patient-centred treatment. Haagen[7] found that clients who were dissatisfied reported lack of empathy and poor ability to handle psychological distress. A qualitative study by Dancet[8] et al found that infertility clients considered the most important aspects of "patient-centred care to be staff attitudes and the relationship with staff, communication, patient involvement and emotional support."

> *At their follow up appointment following a third unsuccessful IVF cycle, Ayden and Arty asked many questions about alternative treatments they had researched on the internet. Whilst the consultant knew about the innovations they were suggesting, he was dismissive of the effectiveness in their case. The couple were not happy with his answer and further questioning from the couple led to the consultant taking a defensive stance. This culminated in Ayden becoming distressed and Arty getting quite angry. They walked out of the clinic*

*saying they would not be back because they did not feel they had been listened to and they would be going to another clinic where they could have this added treatment.*

*Afterwards, the consultant was unhappy that the couple had reacted that way. He did not understand why they had left in anger when he felt he had offered them further treatment which was appropriate for them. If there had been more attention paid to their obvious emotional distress in the session the couple may have felt more listened to and been able to talk through their anxieties, then the outcome may have been different. Using phrases such as, "I can see you have been working hard to research as much as you can and these are the reasons I am not sure this would help you" and, "I see how difficult this has been for you and we want to support you through this" can lead to further open discussion and then a follow-through with the offer of counselling for emotional support.*

*Sometimes, however, couples do need to change clinics as it is one way of exerting control in a situation that leaves them very out of control. Professionals involved in caring through the fertility experience may have to learn to let go in these circumstances.*

Effective communication in a healthcare setting is being able to give clear information about the situation, finding out the clients' expectations, answering questions, offering support and explaining options and decisions. If time is short, setting out the aims of the interchange, a clear idea of the time available and whether there is an opportunity for follow up may make clients feel less rushed or dismissed. Being able to deal with the strong feelings which may arise from the communication, which can be angry or distressed, requires the healthcare professional to be aware and not fearful to be able to manage the responses. Clients may express confusion or denial, anger or aggression. Sometimes clients may appear to trivialise the information given. This may be a way to defend themselves from it. Giving them time and the opportunity to ask questions later helps them to manage the feelings. The communicator must be prepared for all of these outcomes and to find a way to relate to the expectations of the client. A self-assessment checklist Promoting Cultural Diversity and Cultural Competency by Georgetown University[9] reminds staff to consider the environment and their communication styles, as well as their values and attitudes. This could be usefully implemented in all health settings.

## TRAINING IN COMMUNICATION SKILLS

Healthcare staff in training need direct help with communication skills and how to practise them. Much of the training is rightly focused on positive outcomes and the quality of care; but they also need to learn how to communicate when the outcome is not positive and when the client may react with anger, fear or denial. Finding support and a place to reflect on practice is essential for trainees, as well as qualified staff.

Counselling skills will help the practitioner to establish good communication and to offer helpful support. Once they feel comfortable with some of these skills and principles, it will enable them to offer effective communication, even amidst the often-hectic situations in which professionals can find themselves.

## BREAKING BAD NEWS

The nature of obstetrics means that on many occasions, staff will be breaking bad news, sometimes without any time for preparation. Although these are extremely distressing circumstances for all healthcare professionals, their duty of care does encompass this. Those delivering this news will have their own emotional reactions, both to giving the news and to seeing women's reactions after the news has been given. All this can be a devastating experience and healthcare staff can be affected by the strength of their own emotions and reactions.

Much of the information and research into delivering bad news has come from work in the cancer setting. This does not diminish the usefulness of the information in the obstetric situation. The emphasis on learning to be a good and effective communicator is an important part of managing this situation and the topic has not received as much attention as it deserves in the training curriculum. Many clinical situations within maternity care involve the giving of bad news. Some of these include:

- Giving abnormal results to women, including routine investigations and screening results
- Miscarriage
- Terminating a pregnancy
- Intrauterine death
- Stillbirth
- Neonatal poor outcome
- Neonatal death

- Obstetric poor outcome for mother
- Maternal death

Within all these areas there will be specific information the professional will be expected to know. Ensuring they are familiar with the information available for women and their families and to know where to direct them for further information and support is an important part of the role. Being aware that had news can be anything that is unexpected can help. For instance, a diagnosis of Diabetes, can be very frightening and confusing. Bad news is therefore not only related to death but also anything outside of the expectations of the woman, but we won't know what that is unless we know the women very well. It is likely that after breaking bad news the professional will quickly focus on outlining the treatment required. This does not help as the woman may take time to absorb the news and need more time to come to hear and accept this.

There are skills and knowledge that can be learned which help with breaking bad news. These will be very useful when there is a situation that may not be able to be planned for, such as the absence of a heartbeat at scan or routine antenatal appointment

When planning to give bad news, which could be giving results over the phone or in face to face interactions, sufficient time and privacy needs to be allocated. Women reacting to the shock of the news may not absorb the information the first time they receive it and be unable to process it so it may need to be repeated. Leaving space in the conversation allows for reflection. Also, they may be shocked and so unable to process it, so they may need to go away and return at another time to make sense of what they have heard. It is only when they begin to understand the news that they can raise the many questions to which they need answers.

When there is the opportunity to plan the giving of bad news, all the necessary information, including all the relevant results, needs to be gathered before the interaction. Information should be clear and concise and given in a manner the receiver of the information can understand taking into account cultural and religious diversity. Relying on family members to impart delicate and distressing information places a great burden on them.

There is also the risk that they may not have the vocabulary necessary to fully explain this situation. Interpreters are really necessary in this situation as they can choose the words which are appropriate to their native tongue.

Non-verbal communications such as eye-to-eye contact, sitting at the same level as the patient and giving the woman all your attention, help the receiver of the news to feel cared for. Where there is opportunity to prepare, then how you present yourself and the physical space you need requires consideration. Privacy is paramount to a frank and open conversation. Even moving furniture around can make a difference. Sitting at the same level as the client and moving a desk out of the way makes for an easier consultation. Sitting on the same level as the client and at an angle to them is less imposing and offers space to look away if /when eye contact is too challenging.

The health professional will be unsure of the reactions they may have to face, which may feel very confrontational. Shock, anger and sadness are not easy emotions to witness. No professional feels comfortable at these meetings and their anxiety can be very complex. Personal feelings and possibly past experience can get in the way of delivering the news. Medical staff often want to offer factual information such as statistics in an effort to 'give' something to the woman. It helps the member of staff to feel better but may be too much for the woman to hear. Holding off the need to deliver the facts enables the professional to remain focused on the needs of the woman and learn about the implications for that person in her context, culturally, spiritually, and taking into account her religious preferences and within her family setting Monden[10]. This helps to find out what information the woman wants and needs to know. She will begin to ask what she needs to know if she is given the time and space to reach that stage.

Several strategies which offer steps to deliver bad news have been shown to help, SPIKES—A Six-Step Protocol for Delivering Bad News: Application to the Patient with Cancer, Walter F. Baile[11] offers an approach to help when planning to break bad news. Several of the steps in the mnemonic, such as assessing and giving knowledge as appropriate to that woman, being empathetic to her emotional response and planning a forward strategy, all have relevance in pregnancy loss situations. Knowing these can also help when the news that is being broken is unexpected and knowing and applying these steps improves practitioner confidence.

When there is no time to prepare, such as when the professional is giving bad news at a scan appointment, there can be very emotional but different immediate reactions.

> *The sonographer called the bereavement midwife to a scan room, a young woman prostrate on the floor, after receiving the bad news that her baby had died. The staff were very worried and did not know how to manage her very noisy and deep distress. Leaving the scan room was very difficult for her as in her world when she came in all was well and leaving the room would mean recognising that her world had been shattered.*

> *Denial can often be the first reaction to this news and time is needed to allow the news to become real. Some women will need a second scan performed by another member of the team to*

*enable them to have confirmation and help them to adapt to this new situation both in their mind and their body. Gently acknowledging their shock and suggesting a move to another room to consider this news helped the woman to walk out of the room supported by a professional who would be ready to listen and answer questions that arise. It is useful to remember that anyone receiving bad news can react spontaneously outside their usual behaviour patterns which can be a shock to them, their partners/families and the staff present.*

*Selina learned that she had HIV following antenatal testing in the first trimester. The midwife informing her of this result expected shock, anger, tears, or questions at the least. Selina was quiet and reflective and the silence was not easy to experience. The midwife checked Selina's understanding of her situation and still there was no visible reaction. Selina quietly asked what happens next and so that was easy for the midwife to give that information and complete the interview offering appointments and leaflets to read.*

*When the midwife saw Selina again, she was anxious to open up and return to a discussion about how she felt when she was given the news. Selina then broke down and cried with her. She said she had been devastated by the news but in her culture, it was not permissible to show emotions to a stranger, so she had held on to them. She had wanted to cry but, in her silence, she was working very hard at not letting a stranger see her pain. The midwife learned from this experience to expect different reactions. She was able to use the opportunity to raise the issue when they met again in order to better provide care appropriate to her culture, which was helpful to them both.*

The importance of establishing effective communications is clear. When there are language differences, making sure there is an interpreter present is very important and the use of professional interpreters rather than a member of the family is vital. Professionals need to ensure the woman is at the centre of their focus. An interpreter will deliver the information as it has been given, which will enable the woman to ask her questions in her own language. For emotional support and as a second pair of ears, another member of her family can be very helpful.

Not knowing when the skills of breaking bad news may be required can complicate the situation. Those who undertake pregnancy scanning and midwives and obstetricians in clinics are far more likely to be confirming life so are less prepared when there is no heartbeat. In this situation, any healthcare professional can feel at a loss as to how to deliver the information. Using non-medical language, eye to eye contact, tone of voice, touch if this is acceptable to both the giver of the news and the receiver, play an important part in helping at this time. Privacy and dignity will also be important particularly when the news comes whilst the woman is partially undressed as in the scan room or clinic. Whilst this is unexpected for the giver of the information it is shocking to the receiver of the information. Women always remember the words and the manner in which they were told of their loss, this can put more pressure on the professional giving the news.

A small study about how patients felt after they had received bad news raised issues about appropriate communication and patients raised the subject of the numbers of people in the room when news is being broken McCulloch[12]. Cues such as, "I need to talk to this woman, please leave the room" can be given quietly to the extra people. It will alert the woman to a potential problem but that can be explained if handled sensitively and can help prepare her.

There are phrases that can help and be employed when starting the conversation. "I'm afraid it is not good news" and, "The results are not what you were expecting" are two suggestions we have used. Following on with a simple explanation, disbelief and denial are common reactions. Knowledge of stages of loss and attachment theory will give the professionals clues which will enable appropriate support to be offered at this time. Judging what will work at any given time demands sensitivity and reflecting back what you see: "I can see this has been a great shock", is both an observation of the reaction and demonstrates an understanding of the reaction.

> *Returning for a follow-up appointment with the obstetrician following a miscarriage at 21 weeks, Nicky and Simon were expecting to find out why their baby had unexpectedly died. All the test results and the post-mortem had found nothing to point to any definite reason. Their faces looked very puzzled. Taking this as a clue, the doctor said, "You look very puzzled by this". Nicky was first to speak and asked the doctor to repeat what he had said. She gave all the results to them again and waited. This time Simon asked what that meant for them for the future. He had found a way to move the conversation on, but Nicky was still at the 'why?' stage and not ready to consider the future. She crumpled into tears at that point and said, "It must have been my fault, then". For her, there must have been a reason which would in turn have given her hope that it would be*

*different in another pregnancy. Guilt and blame are a response to loss and Nicky was stuck now with these emotions.*

*In these situations, it is natural and easy for the professional to try to give reassurance and hope but this does not help the grieving person. Without the certainty of a better outcome next time Nicky was unwilling to invest in hope. Seeing the devastation in her face, the obstetrician suggested this news was very hard to hear and that Nicky could benefit from having some time with the counsellor to support her through her grief. It was also suggested that she may like to have some sessions with Simon so that they could share feelings. Making sure there is a professional who can respond to the emotional needs of couples at these appointments can guide and help both the obstetrician and the couple to help and support them.*

Breaking bad news in a telephone conversation can be more difficult than face-to-face, partly because there are no visual clues to help with the flow of the delivery. The woman may be at work, so taking care to ensure she has some privacy whilst digesting the information will alert and prepare her. It is still important to allow space for thought but right to use a gentle prompt by repeating that the news is not easy to hear. At the end of the conversation, checking she has someone to speak to about this and helping her manage the immediate work situation helps to ensure she has support after the telephone call ends. Also offering a contact number and name enables a partner to have the conversation continued when they are together again.

*Connie was working with the Specialist Screening Midwife and was contacted by the screening centre with a positive result. As the specialist midwife was not available, she needed to make the phone call to Sarah to tell her the news and arrange for further tests. Connie had listened in to the midwife making these contacts and felt she did have a plan for how to do this. Before she made the call, she looked up information about what the results meant and what further tests could be done. She phoned Sarah, introduced herself and began to explain why she was calling. Her words were met with a tense silence.*

*Connie was not sure what to say next. She had no visible clues to help her now. She carried on with the information she had looked up. It seemed to take a long time until at last Sarah said, "Please could you repeat that". Connie asked where she should start and Sarah said after you said there is a problem with one of your tests. She was then able to slow down with her information and let Sarah tell her what she needed to know.*

*After this phone call Connie reviewed how it had gone with the specialist midwife. Although she had listened into these conversations before, she had not really heard from the woman's point of view and so had been unprepared for Sarah's reaction to her words. Connie had found silence on the phone really unnerving and was not sure whether to prompt or when to prompt.*

What we don't know during silences is what is happening in the mind of the woman. Silence can be a very important part of the conversation. Allowing silence to happen but maybe gently breaking it by using phrases like, "This is a shock for you", and, "I'm here when you can talk" help to encourage further conversation.

In face-to-face conversations, picking up the clues is much easier. For example, shock can be seen in facial expressions, wide eyes, an open mouth, and the body appearing to crumple in on itself as if to ward off the pain. When there is eye contact, sadness is visible in the eyes and a drooping of the mouth; and again, the body folds in, with the arms crossed. These signs can help the professional gauge how to be and what to say to open up conversations such as, "I can see you are shocked … Take your time I am here when you are ready to talk" and, "I can see the sadness in your face".

Simply being with a woman in deep distress is very affecting to professionals and sometimes really difficult to manage. However, encouraging the ventilation of feelings at this time demonstrates to the woman that we are able to offer sensitivity and support and be alongside her through this sad time. In all situations we may simply need to listen to the woman to show her we are with her through this distressing experience.

*When Ayden and Brian had seen the obstetrician concerning the abnormalities found on their 12-week scan they looked very shocked and stunned. The doctor had given a lot of information and set up further scans and appointments, but they seemed reluctant to leave.*

*Taking them into another room, Meg offered them a drink and then sat with them. After a time, they began to talk about what they had heard and how unexpected this morning had been. They came in happy and excited and now their world had fallen apart.*

*Meg was able to offer them space before they faced the world again. She sat with them, offered tissues and when they asked, calmly gave them the information they wanted to know. They made a plan for what would happen next and after an hour they were ready to leave. Later they came back to Meg to tell her how important her intervention had been for them and to thank her for the time she had spent listening to them whilst they tried to make some sense of their situation. Meg was also able to make sure she was with them through the next steps to offer continued support to them both.*

## COMPLICATED COMMUNICATIONS

There are other situations which can add difficulty to effective communications and might sometimes affect the care given. Those who have hearing or sight loss for example will have particular needs such as increased time for appointments and an understanding of how stressful this can be for them. All health carers would benefit from some expert training in managing the inadvertent barriers that prevent effective communication.

## MANAGING ANGER

A natural reaction to bad news is to feel angry and display that emotion verbally and, rarely, physically. A natural reaction to the display of emotions by healthcare staff is to become defensive in the following interchanges. This leads to an increase in the tension in the room and can escalate a difficult situation. There should be no tolerance of any physical display within the team and support to manage aggression made available if it occurs.

Managing any potential difficult situation aims at de-escalating the interactions. Observing the woman/ man and saying what you see: "I can see you are feeling angry", and if it's not obvious, "Can you tell me how are you feeling?" acknowledges this news has engendered a deep reaction. Maintaining eye contact and allowing space for ventilation or just silence allows the woman/ man to offer their take on the situation. Speaking calmly and listening to what is said can give clues to how to work with the anger. This is assertive and can be used in the face of any extreme unusual behaviour. Anything that helps the person to explore and explain rather than to argue will offer the opportunity for de-escalation.

There is also the work of understanding why this particular incident has caused anger. Often, anger comes from fear and being out of control. It could be a repetition of a previous painful experience, but unless explored, it will not be understood.

Healthcare professionals work at solving difficult problems but this may not be possible when pregnancy loss happens, so adopting a listening, caring and supportive approach is more likely to bring about some resolution to anger.

## CARING FOR THE PROFESSIONAL

Just hearing deep distress will touch any healthcare professional. We know that our face will be examined whilst the woman is hoping inside that what is being said is not true (denial) and time is needed to absorb this information. Maintaining silence whilst this occurs is an important part of enabling the woman to make sense of what has been said.

Sometimes after the discussion, staff can be left with feelings they had not anticipated and reminders of their own personal experiences. Seeking support for resolving these feelings is important and a structured reflection with a colleague may help with both the response about the present experience and work out how best to manage in other similar situations.

> *Sitting with Chandra after she had been given bad news at her scan, Gemma was very unsure how to be and what she was meant to do. She felt she had been left alone with Chandra and was unprepared and did not know what to say. Chandra sat in silence and Gemma felt she needed to fill the space. Gemma began to feel quite angry about being in this situation, she felt powerless and very alone. When Chandra moved on to seeing the doctor, Gemma felt very relieved but also very upset. She had found that being with Chandra and witnessing her distress had awakened her own emotions about the pregnancy loss she had experienced a few years ago. No-one knew about this but she had not expected to be challenged in this way.*

Everyone working with families through pregnancy and childbirth will have their own personal stories to tell and these will have some effect on their professional lives either consciously or unconsciously.

Keeping personal information separate can be challenging in some situations but it is usually not helpful to disclose to those in our care. Some may feel they need to do exactly what the professional tells them, even if it conflicts with their thoughts, just to live up to what they perceive will make the professional happy. Others may fear expressing a different point of view as it may impact on their care.

# UNDERSTANDING CULTURAL AND RELIGIOUS RITUALS AROUND LOSS

Differing cultures address rituals and ceremonies around death in different ways and death before birth is connected to spiritual and faith beliefs not always known to the person experiencing the loss of a pregnancy. This only goes to confuse women and faith clergy can certainly help with guiding the way for support. Whilst there are core sets of beliefs around grief and mourning for death and loss, there are also many different rituals and behaviours that are scripted by belief systems around the world.

In order to offer effective support to parents across cultures, it is first important to look at and understand one's own knowledge about your own culture and attitudes towards differing systems. Everyone looks at different cultures through their own cultural viewpoint and when backgrounds differ, there is a challenge to the professional to manage their own personal views. Then the focus will be on assisting the parents to work through their own cultural and/or religious lens.

The experience of pregnancy loss and child death was historically common when pregnancies were many and few contraceptive techniques were available. In older civilisations, loss in pregnancy and childhood was expected and not always seen as significant. Sometimes there were no rituals around this loss and no burial ceremonies. Women were not expected to spend time grieving. Women now have more control over their fertility and have fewer pregnancies. The significance of each of these pregnancies has grown and has become more recognised. This can bring about conflict between the traditional world and the western approach to loss.

The rituals attached to death have become important to the individuals suffering any pregnancy loss whether or not they are connected to religious ceremonies. Everyone mourns for the lost one in both a collective and personal manner. Whilst the collective may include proscribed rituals and ceremonies common to culture and religion, the personal may be experienced differently leading to new individual behaviours and traditions. Those who do not follow any formalised religion may search for something they can attach to, to give them order in the chaos and confusion they are feeling. Rituals can offer comfort in both the collective grief and the personal experience.

Some have beliefs in an afterlife where the soul of the dead person has a journey to complete, either to rest with others as spirits watching over the family or to join ancestors and be born again. This is more clearly defined when individuals having lived a part or the whole of their lives. The situation in pregnancy where the person has not been born alive is less clear and may need some confirmation by the particular faith leaders in order to determine the correct course of events according to that religion and that pregnancy loss. As this may be the individuals' first experience of loss, he/she may not be aware of what practices and rituals his/her religion has for baby loss.

For those who do not have a formalised belief system, finding what works for them is another obstacle they face in their journey through grief. They can build their own rituals around what they feel is needful and meaningful for them and their family.

Working through all this decision-making can be challenging to all healthcare professionals. Firstly, it is wise to make no assumptions based on ethnicity or expressed religion. This subject can be sensitively explored in a non-judgmental way if there are quiet, calm times before delivery. There are common factors to be considered and this can help to raise both the subjects and the support available for decision-making.

## PRIVATE TIME WITH THE BABY

Time after delivery is very precious for those who want to have contact with their baby. Offering them privacy and support may include dressing the baby, taking foot and handprints, taking photos, family visiting and time to be sad and cry.

Contact with the baby is not always what the parents want. In some cultures, women are not expected to see their baby and the men make all the arrangements for the service and the burial. This is usually done with other male members of the family and faith leaders. Roberts[13] et al, looking at social and cultural factors associated with perinatal grief in women in a defined area of India, pointed out that being excluded from ceremonies around the event is balanced by their religious belief that this is done to protect women. If the mother does not have the same faith conviction, this can provoke a religious crisis within the family. Managing this can be a challenge for those healthcare professionals caring for the baby. Keeping in mind the culture of the family and the support the mother will receive from her family and faith will help those who may find this decision difficult to understand.

## ISSUES FOR STAFF

Reflecting and being aware of your own cultural background and attitudes towards other cultures and religions is really important when caring cross-culturally. We all take our past and experiences into our work but to be professional in our approach to women we must work in a non-judgmental way in order to offer sensitive and competent care. The focus of care should always on the needs of the women and their families. We are also reminded that the parents with definite cultural and religious pathways may want to make their own decisions about what they do to honour their baby. In an article for the July 2007 Bulletin for the National Foetal and Infant Mortality Review Program, Jodi Shaefer[14] concluded that, "Whilst it is important to understand the backgrounds and traditions of different racial/ethnic groups it is just as important not to stereotype all people within a particular group".

## DECISION-MAKING

Decision-making is the cognitive process of choosing a belief or action among two or more possibilities. It prompts a final choice but does not necessarily prompt an action. We all make decisions all the time. Some are trivial, such as what to have for lunch or what programme to watch; others are life-changing. We make decisions in different ways depending on our personality, our experience and sometimes social pressure. Some people find it very difficult and endlessly search for more information or advice. They may look on the internet or ask as many people as they can. This may lead to conflicting information or opinions that make it harder to make a choice. Others almost stick a pin in the list. Other people may find it so challenging that they cannot make a choice and will go into a state of denial. 'gut feeling' and intuition also play a part in how we make decisions, although reason may lead to the best outcome.

The decisions that health professionals and their clients make will often be difficult, as they can be life changing. They may also be joint decisions when a couple must find a way to make a choice together. The feeling that one person has influenced the decision unduly may lead to resentment and recrimination. Helping a couple to understand the other's point of view or to reach a decision together may have lasting implications for the relationship.

Most of the theory about how best to make these choices comes from management literature but is appropriate for all difficult decision-making. The steps to take are:

- Identify your goal. What is the purpose of your decision? What is the problem?

- Gather the information you need. This may mean a list of alternatives or information about choices or outcomes. Some people like to have a list of pros and cons. Know when to stop getting information as this can be a way of avoiding the decision. What are the consequences? The final decision may be affected by this both now and in the future

- Make the decision. This may cause anxiety, as it may be that there will be no way back from it. People need to trust their instincts at this point, regarding how they feel and recognise that there are not always perfect choices. Assessing the risk of any decision is based upon the information available.

- Evaluate the decision. This may help with making choices in the future but may also help people to understand why they made that choice at that time, so that they do not struggle with regret or self-recrimination.

## SOCIAL MEDIA

Social media has some great advantages in that people can access information and support easily, can have some questions answered and this may calm anxieties quickly without having to wait for access to a professional.

For people who may be uncertain about asking questions it will help them to find some answers, without fear of seeming 'silly' or ignorant. It also gives them time to look at their own speed and to return to information. Remote, impersonal support may help those who are anxious to speak face to face. However, there are risks. Not all the information is reliable or accurate and scare stories about pregnancy and childbirth abound. Hearing other people's experiences is a double-edged sword: it may offer comfort in shared fears and events, but it may also induce fear and anxiety. It is difficult to help people make judgements about the relevance or accuracy of information on unfiltered social media. We can only warn them that not everything is accurate, and that one person's experience will never be exactly like another's.

Discussing their use of the internet and social media in health issues with two groups, one under 25 years, the other 40 and over, the younger group always chose to look online or on social media first for their information. They were adept at finding their way around the sites and trying to check the information in several ways. They would look for information on NHS sites but would always also look for assessments of the information elsewhere. These women would discuss with friends usually through social media and sometimes look for help on forums of women suffering similar problems.

They did not consider seeking out written information in leaflets or books as this was not the way they look for information. They would only seek medical help if they thought their day to day life was seriously impacted. The older group would also look on the internet but were much more likely to contact a health practitioner face to face. They were more aware of helplines through charities and felt that they could judge the accuracy of information. They rarely accessed written information in the form of leaflets.

The use of the internet and social media will continue to be an increasing area of seeking information and support. Health professionals need to be aware of this and to support people in finding help.

# 8 Endings and New Beginnings

*Attachment and loss; follow-up clinic appointments; endings for the professionals; referrals; new beginnings; preparing for another pregnancy; during another pregnancy.*

Preparing for endings are an important part of the therapeutic process and there are some features that are similar to the ending of the period of mourning after any loss. Holding a public and formal ending, a ceremony/remembrance around death, is very common in many cultures. The timings and format may differ, but their function is for people to come together to acknowledge their sadness at the loss and to celebrate the life lived. When there has been no life outside the womb the marking of the loss for women their partners and their families is concerned with mourning the loss of the hoped- for life. The intensity of emotions around this can be felt by all who attend. For some families it may only be the parents and the close family, others will want to have this space to include friends and sometimes the most immediate healthcare staff who cared for them. There can be little of the celebration aspect and there may be unfinished goodbyes for others attending the service including the healthcare staff.

## ATTACHMENT AND LOSS

Private endings may only be reached when the attachment to the loss diminishes. For the professional engaged with women through this it is useful to consider the attachment theory of Bowlby introduced in the 1960s. Although his concept was originally concerned with mother/child attachment in the early years of life, researchers have now studied prenatal attachment and recognised that the development during the pregnancy is relevant to the continuing bonds after birth. Salehi[1] and Sadheghi[2]. This knowledge can be helpful when understanding the grief experienced when these bonds are severed in an untimely fashion.

Attachment theory is usually connected with loss, as in the child negotiating the separation from the mother. This separation is experienced as a loss by the mother. So the loss of a growing foetus/ baby looked at through this lens, can be seen as an unexpected disruption of the attachment. Feelings are a useful tool to interpret and guide reactions negotiating this loss will be more difficult for those abnormally or unusually attached. Women who have had fertility issues or previous pregnancy losses, may be particularly prone to either insecure or over invested attachments. Knowing this history can help the professional to respond and pay attention to the importance this pregnancy held for the woman. Sensitively asking how they have negotiated through those times before will offer opportunities to explore their coping skills to help them with this experience.

There is no defined time to reach some resolution for this loss. Some women want to disengage, let go and move on quickly, some do not want to stay in the sadness that comes with mourning and move on again quickly but without resolution. Others will take time to go through the tasks of mourning and want to remain attached to their loss. They can fear what will happen if/when they let go. This work happens in the time between appointments with the healthcare professionals and checking out where they are on the grieving process at each appointment will help to determine how best to deliver continuing support.

> *Jesse attended the follow-up clinic 8 weeks after the loss of her baby. She and her partner had consented for the baby to have a post-mortem and they were anxious to hear the results. All the tests that had been performed did not reveal a cause for the death of their baby. Although they had known this was possible, they were both visibly upset at the news. The Consultant thought she was giving good news, i.e. if there was no reason discovered then it was fine to start trying again for another pregnancy. For the couple "no reason" was the worst news they could have. It left them adrift and frightened about starting another pregnancy. Asking what that news meant for them could have opened up the areas the couple had not yet explored and would have given the professional the opportunity to work with the couple towards an understanding of what would help them when they were ready to consider another pregnancy and it would also have given them a supportive framework. Maybe this couple were not ready to let go and needed to take more time to manage their loss. Counselling could be offered as their next step.*

## FOLLOW-UP CLINIC APPOINTMENTS

Managing these appointments provokes many challenges for health professionals and raises the issue of difficult conversations highlighted in the chapter on breaking bad news. It is difficult for healthcare staff to help women and their families when it is the first meeting and they have not been on their journey with them.

Medical staff will want to give information concerning the facts of the loss and can lose sight of the emotional turmoil remaining for the couple. It is never easy to witness displays of emotion, but it is a part of being a professional to be a listener when required.

Both professionals and clients view this appointment with some ambivalence. The couple want to hear about their baby, but they fear getting bad news. The professional wants to get the information across with empathy and sensitivity but the couple may not be known to them which makes responding to their needs difficult.

To be prepared for this appointment, healthcare staff will need to collate all the information they have gathered including any local review of the loss to be able to feedback what has been highlighted by the healthcare team in the weeks after the birth. As an introduction, asking women what they hope to learn from the appointment and what questions they have allows for a better understanding of their needs as to what matters most to the individual or couple.

Attending this appointment may mark the boundary between mourning and accepting the loss. For some, the news they receive will have been of help to them, others may have further investigations to undergo but will still have moved to another place in their loss and feel they are being listened to. Others may not be ready to hear the information and may not feel they are being helped at all.

*After her follow-up appointment with the obstetrician Mona was very unhappy about the outcome. Her baby had been born very early and did not survive labour and birth. The neonatologists had been closely involved during labour and a senior member of the team had spoken with Mona and her partner and attended the birth. This was not the first baby the couple had lost and their anger was felt by all the staff involved in their care. The Specialist Bereavement Midwife had contacted Mona after she went home but Mona was reluctant to take up her offer of support only wanting to know when she would have an appointment to see the obstetrician.*

*At the appointment attended by the Specialist Midwife, Mona and her husband became angry and questioned whether all that could have been done had been done to save her baby. The loss had been reviewed by the maternity team and they had concluded that the measures taken at the time were appropriate. This information did not satisfy either of them.*

*When they walked out of the room still angry, the obstetrician was visibly shaken. He was feeling quite upset and the Specialist Midwife remained to offer support and a debrief. The doctor explained that had felt attacked by the anger in the room and so went into defence mode. This had only resulted in fuelling their anger. There were several things that could have changed the situation. Remaining calm and not reacting in the face of their anger and recognising it was not him they were angry with but their loss could have helped. Listening to their concerns and allowing their expressions of anger without switching into defence may have led to a calmer atmosphere but it is a really difficult thing to do.*

*Acknowledging the anger and using their words to ask what would help them now may be as much as that meeting could have accomplished. It is not always possible to reach an ending where the professional feels they have been able to help the woman. These meetings leave many professionals disheartened. If the professionals engaged in the meeting can recognise that it is not within their power to" make" the woman "feel" better and that offering information to the best of their ability helps women to make their own decisions about how they process the information and what they can do to help themselves.*

*If the information given raises more concerns, then suggesting the couple formally write down their concerns in a letter to senior managers can help them to express these concerns and help them in their journey. This is one way of demonstrating the importance of their wellbeing.*

After any loss at some point the attachment to the loss diminishes. This is a very individual process and can only be accomplished when it is felt that it is OK to let go. Some people may be very anxious about the feelings of loss diminishing as they see this as letting the lost one down, and they need to be helped to feel that this is normal and part of their process of change and moving forward.

Ending brings the opportunity for new beginnings. Reaching this stage is an important milestone for the woman, her family and her wider social network. The future can now be lived even though it is very different.

# ENDINGS FOR THE PROFESSIONALS

Endings for the professionals may not be addressed in the multidisciplinary team. At the end of the shift staff go home with whatever feelings have been awakened to deal with by themselves. Offering a 5 minute debrief at the end of the shift could enable those who wish to, to share their experience with a senior member of the team. The loss may be the first time for some of the staff, or a repeated experience. Both will challenge coping mechanisms. Senior members of the team can offer support and direct those who feel they need more to counselling services.

Healthcare staff develop psychological patterns or coping strategies to manage thoughts, feelings and actions encountered through the challenge of loss in childbearing. There can be long term effects of being with loss which test resilience and if not recognised and managed lead to burnout.

Staff may also be confronted by ethical decisions and dilemmas for both their professional selves and their personal selves. Team members may not have had the experience to manage these issues. They may turn to support from more senior members of the team

Whilst the focus of literature around pregnancy loss is about supporting and caring for women and their families, little has been written about supporting the individuals challenged by managing difficult and traumatic circumstances. The lack of research in this neglected area was highlighted in a study which explored student midwives' experiences for the Royal College of Midwives by Cecilie Begley[3]. She recommended that staff in training should be given clinical experience of caring for bereaved couples with "supervision" and "compassionate support". They should be also offered "debriefing and further support where necessary." This can apply to all healthcare staff during their training or in the first year of practice.

What helps in these situations is early identification of stress and a level of support which is incorporated into clinical practice. In England non-hierarchical supervision for midwives was an effective answer to this, but in systems which value the system ahead of the individual, there is little concentration on these matters. Begley[3] also found student midwives had stories to tell of being shut out of caring for women with loss during their first year of training and then in the next year or after qualifying, needing to care for women with little or no preparation for what to say. They also recounted experiences of lack of support on managing their feelings from the trained staff after looking after women with pregnancy loss.

Generally, coping mechanisms can be divided into active, passive and avoidance. The health worker will employ the coping mechanism that feels most comfortable for them but may not be consciously aware of which they use to respond to these situations. Offering the protected time to the professional to tell the story from their point of view gives the opportunity for the listener to gently explore what feelings were raised.

Allowing space for their grief whilst offering boundaries such as, "We have time for this but it will end" helps to contain their feelings. Just establishing that they are using coping mechanisms and eliciting which they find useful can help them to become more self-aware.

The National Center for Cultural Competence at Georgetown University in the USA has developed a self-assessment checklist for personnel providing services and supports individuals and families affected by Sudden and Unexpected Infant Death (SUID)[4], which provides a very thorough tool that could be used to help review policies and procedures around any pregnancy loss.

Alongside this, the team review of a given situation may bring up professional issues for the individuals involved which may lead to further investigations and they too will need space to address this. Writing responses to investigations and complaints requires some guidance for those new to this situation. Professional bodies have support services both local and national and some have helplines with counselling support for those in need.

## REFERRALS

It can be difficult to let go of a client you have formed a relationship with, particularly through a challenging period of their life. But health professionals are usually not in a position to support the ongoing needs of clients who have experienced losses in pregnancy. This is mainly an issue of time and resources as well as lack of training and sometimes confidence in their ability to help. It is important then to be able to refer clients and their families to people who can give longer term support. There may be counsellors in the healthcare system, GP or hospital setting who can offer sessions during the period of contact or follow up help. Otherwise people may be able to afford private counselling or therapy.

The boundaries of the contact a health professional has with a client may be unclear. Some continue to have contact after the medical intervention has passed, and have formed a bond with them, particularly if they have been with them during a loss. This may make it more difficult to pass the care of the client on to another professional. There is an issue of confidentiality about the information given or received. The client should be made aware of how much information is being given in the referral and should be made aware by the counsellor or therapist what information if any will be given back to the referrer. It can be difficult to recognise that there may be no feedback or follow-up and not knowing what has happened to the client can be very difficult to sit with.

Healthcare professionals need to consider who to refer, when and how the referral should be made. Some clients may ask for help, recognising that all is not well. It may be a challenge to recognise those who are not asking but are considered by staff to need help and are also prepared to accept it and what that help should be. Health professionals need to be able to be clear to the client what support or counselling may be available to them and what that help may offer them so that they have a realistic idea of the process and hoped for outcome. Keeping expectations realistic helps to prevent disappointment about what the helping process might achieve.

Those clients who have a history of mental health problems should have some knowledge of what is available and may be happy to be encouraged to return to the service they have used before. Others may have some reluctance to use the services they think have not been helpful especially when they feel everything has changed for them after a loss. Discussing their needs with empathy and a non-judgmental attitude helps the client and family and others close to them to feel that their needs are recognised. They may need time and encouragement to identify someone whom they trust to make contact with and/or return to therapy or to the mental health services.

Immediately after a loss or a traumatic birth may not be the right time to refer someone, as they may need time to process the experience to understand what they need. If a client or family seems reluctant to engage with the idea of counselling help or other support, the staff may only be able to suggest what help is available and to offer telephone numbers or websites. It is important to check that people feel comfortable with written information or the use of the internet. If they are rejected immediately, these suggestions can always be offered again in the future.

Some women and their partners or families want someone to talk to very soon after a loss. Addressing this with the client, they may be able to tell you if they want help now, and what kind of help they feel would be right for them. Some clients may be reluctant to express their needs or there may be some cultural or family reluctance to seek outside help. Spending time with the woman alone may help her to express her needs. It may only be possible to offer written information and signposts to support groups or the major charities.

Where there are languages spoken other than English, NHS 111 or some of the major charities offer help. Giving contact numbers or email address which can be kept for when they feel ready to make use of it may be all that is possible, but still feel that the staff are offering something and the family understand that their feelings are being acknowledged. If there is a counsellor or midwife or nurse with counselling qualifications a name can be very reassuring, even if the client does not make contact immediately. For those in a position to pay, lists of accredited counsellors are available from BACP (see Resources section).

## NEW BEGINNINGS: PREPARING FOR ANOTHER PREGNANCY

The psychological impact of loss will continue into thoughts of another pregnancy. There will be questions about when and how to cope with the inevitable anxiety. Pregnancy after loss is not like pregnancy before loss. Every milestone from the pregnancy test onward feels different. Knowing the right time to become pregnant again is a very individual decision. Too soon, and the feelings of loss can be re-ignited conversely waiting for a long time may result in fertility problems for the woman or increase her fear.

Parents may feel under pressure to try again and may be asked by well-meaning people when they will have another or suggest that this might make them feel better about the loss. For some it may not be possible for medical reasons. Others may be too anxious to contemplate another pregnancy.

*Jody and Jess revealed at their follow up visit that they had not resumed sexual relations following their difficult birth experience. The reluctance to have sex again was not coming from Jody but from Jess. They were attending counselling to explore the reasons for his reluctance and came together to the sessions. Jess had witnessed what he experienced as shocking things during the birth of their now healthy baby. He explained it had left him with many feelings he had not been able to dispel.*

*He described seeing the doctors handling the private parts of his wife's anatomy and cutting her as horrific and shocking. He could still see it all happening in his mind. This was affecting him whenever intimacy was suggested or initiated by his wife. Hearing this reduced them both to tears but they did not reach out to support each other.*

*He also said he felt very responsible for the part he had played in making the pregnancy which led to the birth. He did not want to ever put his wife in this situation again so not having sex was his way of avoiding it. After expressing all this emotion, he said he felt better now that it was all out of him. They both needed time to grieve for the loss of the labour they had envisioned and the loss of control they both felt throughout the delivery. Work could then commence on addressing and managing his reactions and then his fears and anxieties about getting pregnant again. Psychosexual work helped them to re-establish their sex life with intimacy exercises and talk therapy. When it was right for them to try for another pregnancy, they asked for support through the pregnancy from the obstetric team. They took his worries seriously and involved him in each decision.*

Many fears will accompany even thinking about another pregnancy. The partners may not agree on having a further pregnancy or the timing. There will be a loss of confidence in having a healthy pregnancy and baby. Also, the fear of repetition alongside the fear of the pain and grieving involved if loss happens again makes starting again fraught with anxiety. Patients pregnant through assisted conception have the added complication of needing more treatment without the promise of success.

Often there is little contact with healthcare professionals through this time. GPs may be approached and offer guidance about the physical aspects and health information. They can be a source for information about risks, the support available, and possible referral to a genetic specialist.

Pre-conceptual advice concerning smoking/exercise etc may help them to feel they can do something to help the situation but there is little support for those who need time for reflection and discussion.

## DURING ANOTHER PREGNANCY

The term 'rainbow babies' has been coined for babies born after loss and it may be useful for the professionals to have a defined pathway of care for these pregnancies. There are a number of issues that those caring for women and their families in this pregnancy need to be aware of because there are changed expectations to be managed.

Contact with the healthcare team may be very early and, depending on the history, women may want early scans to see their tiny growing embryo as soon as possible. Returning to the place where the pregnancy loss was first diagnosed is daunting for the woman and can place extra demands on the EPU staff, tact, empathy, understanding and gentle support will help to alleviate anxiety.

Other women may avoid contact or book quite late in this pregnancy, this can be of concern to the healthcare team who will want to ensure all the tests, scans and examinations are completed in a timely manner. Understanding that it is the overwhelming fear that it could happen again that may have made them delay can help the professionals to manage this sensitively. For the woman, taking it day by day may be the only way to manage this stressful time.

Another way of managing through this difficult time is to distance yourself from the pregnancy. How can you let yourself fall in love with this one when the other one disappeared? In other words, it may be the final step in the grieving process in accepting the past and letting it go. It is a way to keep the emotions safe and not engaged, which can have other interpretations for the professionals. Acknowledging that the woman may need to suppress her feelings in order to negotiate the pregnancy can relieve the woman for any guilt feelings she may have at not being excited about this pregnancy. Women can be disappointed that they do not feel the happiness and joy they thought they would. Health professionals can help by understanding that what has happened in their past will have a bearing on this pregnancy and simply ask, "How are you feeling about this pregnancy?" and, "How can we best support you?".

Much of this also applies to the partners who look on and worry, often silently. They can feel powerless and unable to address their worries. Whilst supporting their partner offers a way to help, they may not feel at all in control themselves. Professionals could include them in discussions in the early stages and offer support to them too. Much of the anxiety experienced by them both is indicative of a need to feel and stay in control.

When the reaction to being pregnant is not happiness, others around the woman may wonder at this. The reactions of other family members may increase or reduce any anxiety, and the woman and her partner may delay sharing their news until at least the first 12 weeks are over. They may change their decisions about routine tests and more information may be required including referral for a specialised opinion.

The question arises, "can this pregnancy be enjoyed at all?" There will be degrees of anxiety for women up to and around previous loss. It may then change, or other worries take over so some women may go through the whole pregnancy needing a great deal of emotional support to manage their anxiety. Counselling can be of help to individuals by holding onto their worries as they negotiate through the different stages of this new pregnancy.

# 9: In Conclusion

In researching and writing this book and reflecting on our own practice, we understand that healthcare professionals do want to communicate effectively and offer the best care to their clients. They need resources, support and training in managing situations where they are "lost for words". We hope we have helped a little and offered signposts along the way to provide further information and support.

# RESOURCES
# Where to find support, guidelines and information

## CHARITIES

There are charities at international, national and local levels which offer support for loss in pregnancy at all stages. They complement statutory services offering: the raising of awareness for patients, families and professionals; promoting good practice, individual and group support by telephone, online and, in some cases, face-to-face; written advice and information; signposting other services and research. They use employed staff and volunteers to whom they offer training. Coverage across countries varies but the use of the internet means that most people can access some level of support and advice.

The main national charities in the area of pregnancy loss in the UK are:

### The Miscarriage Association - miscarriageassociation.org.uk

Offers leaflets in a range of languages and help on the telephone and online for women and their families who have suffered a loss by miscarriage, molar pregnancy or ectopic pregnancy. Their website offers information, guidance and support, including for those considering another pregnancy and specific help for young people and their partners.

### The British Pregnancy Advice Service (BPAS) - bpas.org

Offers help in considering an abortion, finding a clinic and post-abortion support. Their website has a resources section for professionals, which includes information, training and details of their research.

### The Ectopic Pregnancy Trust - ectopic.org.uk

Supporting people who experienced an early pregnancy complication and the healthcare professionals who care for them.

### Molar Pregnancy Support and Information - molarpregnancy.co.uk

Provides information and support to women who are currently or have previously suffered from a molar pregnancy.

### ARC (Antenatal Results and Choices) - arc-uk.org

Offers support and information to parents throughout antenatal testing and results, and where there has been a diagnosis of foetal anomaly.

### TOMMY's tommys.org

Funds research into miscarriage and stillbirth. They run clinics, research centres, a pregnancy information service and a support line.

### The Stillbirth and Neonatal Death Charity SANDS - sands.org.uk

Operates throughout the UK offering support to anyone affected by the loss of a baby. They have a helpline, support groups and an online community. They offer support for professionals and are involved with education and research. They are currently translating several of their leaflets into other languages and have set up an app for parents and families.

### MAMA Academy - mamaacademy.org.uk

Helps to empower parents, educate healthcare professionals and generally raise awareness of the issues around stillbirth and early infant mortality.

### BLISS - bliss.org.uk

Offers a helpline and email support, with volunteers who support parents locally, as well as volunteer assessors who evaluate family-centred care in neonatal units. Their vision is that every baby born prematurely or sick in the UK has the best chance of survival and quality of life.

### The Birth Trauma Association - birthtraumaassociation.org.uk

Supports women who suffer birth trauma and also PTSD related to birth trauma.

### Child Bereavement UK - 0800 0288840

Offers support to families and education to professionals when a baby or child dies or is dying.

### TAMBA - tamba.org.uk

Supports those who have lost a twin.

There are also local charities offering encounter group support, apps or online help. The main organisations offer help to Black, Asian and Minority Ethnic clients and there are also some local organisations that offer specific help, especially with language needs. These can be reached online. Full lists of charities can be found via the main organisations, or by searching more specifically.

The larger charities like the Miscarriage Association report increased use of social media, including more people posting on Facebook pages.

Mumsnet has surveyed its users on various topics including their experiences of miscarriage.

There are also many organisations offering help with making memory items such as plaster for hand and footprints, supplying these items for use in hospitals and to women and their families. We cannot recommend any of these websites or organisations, so individuals will need to do their own research and assess their value by reading what they offer.

Charities concerned with Mental Health include:

### MIND - mind.org.uk

The Mental Health Charity offers information and support about mental health and treatments nationally and locally.

### CRUSE- Cruse.org.uk

Face-to-face, telephone and online services which offer support, advice and information for children, young people and adults when someone dies.

### The National Eating Disorders Association -nationaleatingdisorders.org

Offers information, support and understanding to people with eating disorders and their families. This is a US Helpline.

### Alcoholics Anonymous (AA) - 0800 9177650

A self-help group support for those wanting help to stop drinking.

### Narcotics Anonymous (NA) - 0300 9991212

Self-help user-led groups supporting those who want to stop using drugs.

### Addiction - www.addiction.org.uk

Working in the community with adults and young people with drug and alcohol problems.

### Drinkline -     0300 1231110

Telephone support for people with alcohol problems.

Full lists of charities can be found via the main organisations, or by searching more specifically.

# OFFICIAL GOVERNMENT ORGANISATIONS

There are official government resources for guidance and information:

### Epicure.ac.uk

Population based studies of survival and later health status in extremely premature infants.

### MMBRACE npeu.ox.ac.uk

A national collaborative programme of work involving the surveillance of mothers and babies who die. Reducing the risk through audits and confidential enquiries across the UK

### The National Institute for Health and Care Excellence - nice.org.uk

Offers up to date policies, procedures, guidance and advice on quality standards. It has a series of information sites and latest guidance on treatment and practice. Their website also offers journals and databases.

### NHS Choices - nhs.uk

Offers information on a wide range of conditions and on social care. Scotland, Wales and Northern Ireland also have NHS Choices sites, with some specific information.

# PROFESSIONAL ORGANISATIONS

These professional bodies offer regulation, membership, accreditation, and some information, education and support.

### The Association of Early Pregnancy Units - aepu.org.uk

Offers support and resources to help patient choice and to maintain standards in Early Pregnancy Units.

### The Nursing and Midwifery Council - nmc.org.uk

Regulates nurses and midwives in the UK. They set standards, hold a register, indicate quality assured education and investigate complaints. They also publish reports, policy documents and research papers.

### The Royal Colleges of Nursing and Midwifery - rcn.org.uk/rcm.org

Offers support and have bereavement networks for midwives, nurses and students. They also offer online training modules on bereavement care.

### Skills for Health

Offers online training in awareness of mental health and communication, as well as many others.

### The Royal College of Obstetricians and Gynaecologists - rcog.org.uk

Aims to improve the care of women, encourage research and education, publish guidelines and information leaflets. They provide continuing professional development for doctors working in the specialty.

**Obstetric Ultrasound - radiologyinfo.org**

An American group offering information about obstetric ultrasound to pregnant women

The above and other professional organisations are working together with support organisations and charities in developing a National Bereavement Care Pathway for England backed by the government which aims to overcome inequalities and improve the quality of services with measurable outcomes for parents and professionals.

**The British Association for Counselling and Psychotherapy (bcap.co.uk)**

Offers information, support and accreditation for counsellors and psychotherapists, which ensures a level of training and practice, as there is no regulatory body for therapy. Its website offers a list of accredited therapists in all regions.

Training in counselling is offered by universities and colleges throughout the country at all levels. There are also some online training programmes in most English-speaking areas. Those interested should check that it can lead to accreditation and look for the concepts and skills that it offers.

**The United Kingdom Council for Psychotherapy (psychotherapy.org.uk)**

Offers training and accreditation for psychotherapists.

Further information about all of these is available online.

# OTHER RESOURCES

The Center for Disease Control and Prevention in the USA has some online and Facebook linked information around loss in pregnancy and childbirth, as does The Office on Women's Health.

There are online lists of support groups for pregnancy loss in Canada.

Pregnancy Loss Australia offers support and guidance on miscarriage, stillbirth and infant loss.

All these are accessible online.

# References

## INTRODUCTION

1.  N. Brier. *Grief Following Miscarriage: A comprehensive review.* Journal of Women's Health (3). 2008.

## CHAPTER 1

1.  J Bowlby. *Attachment and Loss.* Vol 1.Separation Vol 11. Tavistock. 1975.
2.  E. Kubler-Ross. *On Death and Dying.* Tavistock. 1970.
3.  J. Bowlby. *Attachment and Loss.* 1980.
4.  C. Murray-Parkes. *Bereavement: Studies of grief in adult life.* Penguin. 1976.
5.  G. Engel. *Is Grief a Disease? A Challenge for Medical Research.* Psychosomatic Medicine. 1961.
6.  W. Worden. *Grief Counselling and Grief Therapy.* Routledge. 1992.
7. J. Savage. 'Mourning Unlived Lives'. Chiron Pub. 1989.

## CHAPTER 2

1.  A. Jutel. *Death Before Birth.* Perspectives in Biology and Medicine. 49 (2). 2006.
2.  B. McCreight. *Grief: Ignored narratives of loss from a male perspective.* Sociology of Health and Illness. March, 2014.
3.  E. Peel and R. Ellis. 'Silent Miscarriage and Deafening Herteronormativity: A British experiential and critical feminist account'.
4.  Emma Robertson Blackmore, *et al. Previous Prenatal Loss as a Predictor of Perinatal Depression and Anxiety.* British Journal of Psychiatry. 2011.
5.  A. Guillaume and C. Rossier. *Abortion Around the World: A review of legislation, measures, trends and consequences.* Population. Vol 73. 2018.
6.  H. Lindemann. *Holding On and Letting Go: The social practice of personal identities.* Oxford Scholastic Online. 2014.
7.  R. Hess. *Dimensions of Women's Long Term Post-abortion Experience.* American Journal of Maternal/Child Nursing May. 2004.
8.  A. Lipp. *Termination of Pregnancy: A review of psychological effects on women.* Nursing Times. January, 2009.
9.  A. Broen, T. Moum, A. Sejersted-Bodtker & O. Ekeberg. *Predictors of Anxiety and Depression following Pregnancy Termination: A five-year follow-up study.* Journal of Obstetrics and Gynaecology, Scandinavia. Vol 85. 2006.
10. C. Cozzarelli. *Mental Models of Attachment and Coping with Abortion.* Journal of Personality and Social Psychology. Vol 74. 1998.

11. B. Bonevski and J. Adams. *Termination of Pregnancy: A review of the psychological effects on women.* Nursing Times. 2001.

12. G. Zolese & C. V. Blacker. *The Psychological Complications of Therapeutic Abortion.* British Journal of Psychiatry. 1992.

13. Gilchrist, P.et al. *Termination of Pregnancy and Psychological Morbidity.* British Journal of Psychiatry. August, 1995.

14. Clare A W, Tyrrell J. *Psychiatric Aspects of Abortion.* Irish Journal of Psychological Medicine, Volume 11, Issue 2, June 1994 P 92-98.

15. M Fine-Davis. *Psychological effects of Abortion on Women a review of the literature.* University College Dublin Crisis Pregnancy Report, Dec 2007.

16. N L Stotland, *et al. Antenatal risk Factors for Postpartum Depression, a synthesis of literature.* Academic Press NY 1977.

17. Robbins. *Out of Wedlock Abortion and Delivery, the Importance of the Male Partner.* Social Problems, 1984.

18. J Farren, *et al. Post Traumatic Stress, Anxiety and Depression following Miscarriage and Ectopic Pregnancy: A prospective cohort study.* British Medical Journal 2016, BMJ Open.

19. Guerra Benute *et al. Depression, stress and guilt are linked to the risk of suicide associated with ectopic pregnancy.* Medical Express 2016 open access.

20. Catherine Chojenta *et al. History of Pregnancy Loss Increases the Risk of Mental Health in Subsequent Pregnancies but Not in the Postpartum.* 2014 open access.

21. Valentina E Di Mattei, Letizia Carnelli. *An Investigative Study into Psychological and Fertility Sequelae of Gestational Trophoblastic Disease: The Impact on Patients' Perceived Fertility, Anxiety and Depression: PLoS One.* 2015 Jun1. doi; 10.1371/journal.pone.01283354.

22. Rodney W Petersen, Kim Unga, Cynthia Holland, Julie A Quinlivan. *The impact of molar pregnancy on psychological symptomatology, sexual function, and quality of life.* Gynecological 2005.

23. Lari Wenzel, Ross Berkowitz, Sharon Robinson, Marilyn Bernstein, Donald Goldstein. *The Psychological, Social, and Sexual Consequences of Gestational Trophoblastic Disease.* Gynecologic Oncology 46.(1) 74-81 1992.

24. Jane Ireson, Georgina Jones, Matthew C Winter, Stephen C Radley, Barry W Hancock, John A Tidy. *Systematic Review of Health-Related Quality of Life and Patient-Reported Outcome Measures in Gestational Trophoblastic Disease: a Parallel Synthesis Approach.* The Lancet Oncology 2018.

25. Sheryl S Heller and Charles H Zeanah. *Attachment Disturbances in Infants Born Subsequent to Perinatal Loss; A pilot study.* 20 (2), 188-199 Infant Mental Health Journal 1999.

26. Corbett, Owen and Kruger, quoted in *Emotional Care for women who Experience Miscarriage,* R Evans, Nursing Standard 2012

27. Chan Moon Fai, D Arthur. *Nurses' attitudes towards perinatal bereavement care.* Journal of Advanced Nursing 2001.

28. R Murphy & J Merrell. *Negotiating the Transition: caring for woman through the experience of early miscarriage.* Journal of Clinical Nursing, June ,2009.

29. C Roehrs *et al.* *Caring for Families Coping with Perinatal Loss.* Journal of Obstetric, Gynaecological and Neonatal Nursing, November, 2008.

# CHAPTER 3

1. L. Regan and R. Rai. *Epidemiology and the Medical Causes of Miscarriage: Best Practice and Research in Clinical Obstetrics and Gynaecology.* Vol. 14, Issue 5, Pages 839-854.October 2000.

2. R.J. Benzie et al. *How much do women know about first trimester ultrasound and serum screening?* ASUM Ultrasound Bulletin 7(3):13-4. 2004.

3. A. Ledward. *Pregnant Women's Experiences of Screening for Foetal Abnormalities According to NICE Guidelines: How should midwives communicate information?* Evidence Based Midwifery 15(4): pp. 112-119. 2017.

4. H.Skirton and O. Barr. I*nfluences of Antenatal Screening for Down Syndrome: A review of the literature.* RCM Evidence Based Midwifery. 20

5. UK National Screening Committee Guidelines: *Antenatal screening Guide to 2018/19 screening specifications.*

6. V. Davies *et al.* *Psychological Outcome in Women Undergoing Termination of Pregnancy for Ultrasound--detected Foetal Anomaly in the First and Second Trimesters: A pilot study.* Ultrasound in Obstetrics and Gynaecology. Vol. 25, Issue 4. 2005.

7. A. Kersting *et al.* *Psychological Impact on Women after Second and Third Trimester Termination of Pregnancy Due to Foetal Abnormalities versus Women After Preterm Birth – a 14-month Follow-up Study.* Archives of Women's Mental Health. August, 2009.

8. B. Nazarre *et al.* *Adaptive and Maladaptive grief responses following TOPFA; actor and partner effects of coping strategies.* Journal of Reproductive and Infant Psychology. Volume 31, Issue 3, pages 257-273: 2013.

9. M C A White-Van Mourik *et al.* *The psychosocial sequelae of a second-trimester termination of pregnancy for fetal abnormality.* Prenatal diagnosis Volume 12, issue 3 Pages 189-204 March 1992.

10. Ekelin M, Crang-Svalenius E, Dykes AK. *A qualitative study of mothers' and fathers' experiences of routine ultrasound examination in Sweden.* Midwifery. pp 335-44.2004 Dec, 2004

11. Jo Garcia. Leanne Bricker, Jane Henderson, Marie-Anne Martin, Miranda Mugford, Jim Nielson, Tracy Roberts. *Women's views of pregnancy ultrasound : A systematic review.* Birth - Issues in Perinatal Care : Volume 29, Issue 4,

12. Lynne Gillam, Dominic Wilkinson,Vicki Xafis David Isaacs *Decision-making at the borderline of viability: Who should decide and on what basis?* Journal of Paediatrics and Child Health Volume 53. Issue 2 Pages 105-111: February 2017.

13. Ali M Nadroo. *Ethical dilemmas in decision making at limits of neonatal viability.* Journal of The Islamic Medical Association of North America Volume 43: Pages 189 -192 Dec 2012.

14. RCOG Scientific Impact Paper No 41. *Perinatal Management of Pregnant Women at the Threshold of Infant Viability (The Obstetric Perspective).* Feb 2014.

15. British Association of Perinatal Medicine. *The Management of babies born Extremely Preterm at less than 26 weeks of gestation: A Framework for Clinical Practice at the Time of Birth.* Archives of Diseases of Childhood, Oct 6, 2008

# CHAPTER 4

1. Office of National Statistics Stillbirth data 2017

2. WHO: *Maternal, newborn, child and adolescent health* 2016

3. WHO *Improve Data by setting a standardization system for classifying stillbirths and neonatal deaths.* 2018

4. *Every Woman Every Child . Global Strategy for Women's, Children's, and Adolescents' Health (2016-2030)*

5. Jane Arezina. *What training in difficult news delivery do sonographers have and what impact do sonographers who regularly deliver difficult news think this has on their levels of wellbeing and burnout? A CoRIPs funded study.* (Powerpoint presentation) BMUS Obstetric Study Day, 13 October 2017. Birmingham Events and Conference Centre. By kind permission.

6. Late *Intrauterine Fetal Death and Stillbirth.* RCOG Green Top Guideline . 55 2010

7. *Nice Antenatal and Postnatal Mental Health; Clinical Management and Service Guideline.* Updated 2018

8. Beate, Andre *et al. Culture of silence: Midwives', obstetricians' and nurses' experiences with perinatal death.* Clinical Nursing Studies Vol 4 No 4 58-65 2016

9. Can Cemal Cingi *et al. Will communication strategies in patient relations improve patient satisfaction?* The International Journal of Communication and Health No 7 2015 40-45

10. D Nuzum, S Meaney, K O'Donoghue, *The impact of stillbirth on consultant obstetrician gynaecologists: a qualitative study.* Royal College of Obstetricians and Gynaecologists. Published online March 2014

11. Sonya Wallbank, Noelle Richardson. *Midwife and nurse responses to miscarriage, stillbirth and neonatal death: a critical review of qualitativ*e Evidence Based Midwifery: RCM 2008

12. Cecily Begley. *I cried ... I had to ... Sudent Midwives' Experience of Stillbirth, Miscarriage and Neonatal Death.* Evidence Based Midwifery. RCM 2009

13. P Hughes, P Turton. E Hopper, CDH Evans. *Assessment of guidelines for good practice in psychosocial care of mothers after stillbirth: a cohort study.* The Lancet Vol 360 Issue 9327 , P 114-118 13th July 2002

14. Kerstin Eriandsson, Jane Warland, Joanne Cacciatore, Ingela Radestad. *Seeing and holding a stillborn baby: Mother's feelings in relation to how their babies were presented to them after birth - Findings from an on- line questionnaire.* Midwifery Vol 29, Issue 3 , P 246-250 , March 2013

15. David Kessler *et al. Debriefing in the Emergency Department After Clinical Events: A Practical Guide.* Annals of Emergency Medicine 1-9: 2014

16. Elizabeth S Draper, Ian D Gallimore, Jennifer J Kurinczuk, Peter W Smith, Thomas Boby, Lucy K Smith, Bradley N Manktelow on behalf of the MBRRACE-UK collaboration. *MBRRACE-UK Perinatal Mortality Surveillance Report UK*

*Perinatal Deaths for Births from January to December 2016.* Summary Report . 2017

17. Judy Richards *et al. Mothers' Perspectives on the perinatal loss of a co-twi: a qualitative study.* BMC Pregnancy and Childbirth, 2015 15(1):143

18. Nancy Segal. *Loss of a twin is a devastating life event:* psychology today, posted Jul 27, 2009

19. NICE Clinical Guideline 129 2011

20. Knight M *et al* (Eds.) on behalf of MBRRACE-UK. *Saving Lives, Improving Mothers' Care - Lessons learned to inform maternity care from the UK and Ireland Confidential Enquiries into Maternal Deaths and Morbidity 2014-16.* Oxford: National Perinatal Epidemiology Unit, University of Oxford 2018

21. Rosemary Mander. *When the Professional gets personal - the midwife's experience of the death of a mother.* Evidence Based Midwifery: Royal College of Midwives 2009

22. Rhoda Suubi Muliira, Marie C Bezuidenhout. *Occupational exposure to maternal death: Psychological outcomes and coping methods used by midwives working in rural areas.* Midwifery Journal Volume 31 Issue 1 184-190 2015

23. Hong Zhu *et al. The Effect of Maternal Death on the Health of the Husband and Children in a Rural Area of China: A Prospective Cohort Study.* PLoS ONE 11(6)

24. Rachel Collins, What is the purpose of debriefing wo25men in the postnatal period. RCM Evidence Based Midwifery 2009

25. Bastos M, Furuta M, Small R, McKenzie-McHarg K, Bick D: Debriefing interventions for the prevention of psychological trauma in women following childbirth: Cochrane Database of Systematic Reviews 2015 Issue 4

26. Ayers S, Claypool J, and Eagle A; *What happens after a difficult birth? Postnatal debriefing services.* British Journal of Midwifery 14 (3) 2006, 157-161

27. Cathy Rowan, Debra Brick: *Postnatal debriefing Interventions to prevent Maternal Mental Health Problems after Birth: Exploring the Gap Between the Evidence and UK Policy and Practice: Worldviews on Evidence- based.* Nursing Volume 4 Issue 2 97-105

28. Kersting A, Dolemeyer R, Steinig J ,Walter F, Kroker K, Baust K, Wagner B. *Brief Internet based intervention reduces post -traumatic stress and prolonged grief in parents after the loss of a child during pregnancy: a randomised control trial.* Psychotherapy Psychosomatics; 82(6):372-81. Epub 2013

29. Gold Katherine J, Johnson Timothy. *Mothers at Risk: Maternal Health Outcomes After Perinatal Death.* Obstetrics and Gynecology 123 Suppl 1:6S · May 2014

30. Jennifer L Huberty *et al. When a Baby Dies. A Systematic Review of Experimental Interventions for Women after Stillbir*th. Reproductive Sciences, 24(7), 967–975. 2016

31. Health and Safety Executive. *Providing support after an incident* 2013

# CHAPTER 5

1. Howard. 2014 article in the British Journal of Psychiatry Reviewed by the RCM 2018 *"One in four pregnant women have mental health problems."*

2.  I. Brockington. *Motherhood and Mental Health* Oxford 1996

3.  S Prady, K Pickett, E Petherick, S Gillbody. *Evaluation of Ethnic Disparities in the detection of depression and anxiety in primary care during the maternal period.* Combines analysis of routine and cohort data. British Journal of Psychiatry May 2016

4.  N Gavin *et al. Perinatal Depression: a systematic review of prevalence and incidence.* Obstetric Gynaecology November 2005

5.  J Evans, J Heron, H Francomb, S Oke, J Golding. *Cohort Study of depressed mood during pregnancy and after childbirth.* British Medical Journal, April 2001

6.  M Norhayati, N Hazlina, A Asrenee,W Wan Emilin. *Magnitude and risk factors for postpartum symptoms: A literature review.* Journal of Affective Disorders, April 2015

7.  RCOG & MMHA Only 7% of women with mental health problems during pregnancy are referred to specialist care 2017

8.  K L Wisner *et al. Postpartum Depression: a Disorder in Search of a Definition.* Archives of Women's Health, Feb 2010

9.  E Russell, J Fawcett, D Mazmanian. *Risk of obsessive-compulsive disorder in pregnant and postpartum women: a meta-analysis.* Journal of Clinical Psychiatry, April 2013

10. O Vesga-Lopez, C Blanco, K Keyes, M Olfson, B Grant, D Hasin. *Psychiatric disorders in pregnant and postpartum women in the US.* Archive of General Psychiatry, July 2008

11. S Ayers, A Eagle, H Waring . *The effects of childbirth related post-traumatic disorder on women and their relationships: a qualitative study.* Psychology, Health and Medicine vol 11 2006

12. P Yildiz, S Ayers, L Phillips. *The prevalence of post-traumatic disorder in pregnancy and after birth: A systematic review and meta-analysis.* Journal of Affective Disorders January 2017

13  J Farren *et al. Post-traumatic Stress, Anxiety and Depression Following Miscarriage or Ectopic Pregnancy.* BMJ Nov 2016

14. M W Otto, J A J Smits, H E Reese. *Cognitive behavioural therapy for the treatment of anxiety disorders.* The Journal of Clinical Psychiatry 65 2019

15. F Walsh. *Family resilience: a developmental systems framework.* European Journal of Developmental Psychology March 2016

16. A Valiente-Gomez, A Moreno-Alcazar, D Treen, C Cedron, F Colom, V Perez and B Amann. *EMDR beyond PTSD: a systematic Literature Review.* Frontiers in Psychology August 2017

17. A Easter, A Bye , E Taborelli, F Corfield *et al. Recognising the symptoms: how common are eating disorders in pregnancy.* European Eating Disorder Review July 2013

18. H Watson *et al. Psychosocial Factor associated with bulimia nervosa during pregnancy an internal validation study.* International Journal of Eating Disorders, 2014

19. N Troop, J Treasure. *Psychosocial factors in the onset of eating disorders: Responses to life events.* British Journal of Medical Psychology July 2011

20. H Watson, L Torgerson, S Zerwas *et al. Eating Disorders, Pregnancy and the Postpartum Period: findings from the Norwegian mother and child cohort study.* Norway Epidemiol January, 2014

21. L M Howard *et al The general fertility rate in women with psychotic disorders.* Am Journal of Psychiatry, 2002

22. L Lydsdottir. *The Maternal Health Characteristics of pregnant with depressive symptoms identified by the Edinburgh Postnatal Depression Scale.* Journal of Clinical Psychiatry, 2014

23. E Robertson et al. *Risk of puerperal and non-puerperal recurrence of illness following puerperal psychosis.* British Journal of Psychiatry March, 2005

24. U. Valdimarsdottir *et al. Psychotic illness in first time mothers with no previous hospitalizations.* P LoS Medicine Feb 2009

25. R Sherwood. *Substance Misuse in Early Pregnancy and relationship to fetal outcome.* European Journal of Pediatrics, 1999

26. S Williamson *et al. Determination of the prevalence of drug misuse by meconium analysis.* Archives of Disease in Childhood, 2006

27  J Glanz & J Woods. *Obstetrical Issues in Substance Abuse.* Pediatric Annals, 1991

28. A Forray. *Perinatal Substance Use: a prospective evaluation of abstinence and relapse.* Alcohol and Drug Dependency (US 2015)

29. University of Bristol L Mamluk & L Zuccolo for MRC and others pub. BMJ Open access bmjopen@bmj.com 2017

30. S Popova, S Lange, C Probst *et al. WEstimation of national, regional, global prevalence of alcohol use during pregnancy and Fetal Alcohol Syndrome: a systematic review and meta-analysis.* Lancet Global Health, March 2017

31. S Brooks, C Gerada, T Chalder. *Review of literature on the mental health of doctors: are specialist services needed?* Journal of Mental Health, January 2011

32. G Mark & A Smith. *Occupational stress job characteristics. Coping and the mental health of nurses.* British Journal of Health Psychology 2011

33. S Moll, A Frolic & B Kay. *Investing in compassion exploring mindfulness as a strategy to enhance personal relationships in healthcare practice.* Journal of Hospital Administration vol 4 no.6 2015

34. C Joan-Simpson, F Pilkington, C MacDonald *et al. Nurses experience of grieving when there is a perinatal death.* Sage Open April 2013

35. S Shapiro, S Astin, J Bishop,R Scott, M Cordova. *Mindfulness Based Stress Reduction for health care professionals : results from a randomised trial.* International Journal of Stress Management May 2005

36. J Saunders & S Valente. *Nurses' Grief.* Cancer Nursing 1994

37. V Downey, M Bengiamin, L Heuer, N Juhl. *Dying Babies and associated stress in NICU Nurses.* Neonatal Network 1995

38. P Marris. *The Politics of Uncertainty.* 1996 Routledge

39. S Wallbank & N Robertson. *Predictors of staff distress in response to professionally experienced miscarriage, stillbirth and neonatal loss: a questionnaire study.* British Journal of Nursing Studies, 2013

40. K Doka (ed). *Disenfranchised Grief: recognising hidden sorrow.* 2001, New York

# CHAPTER 6

There are no references in this chapter.

# CHAPTER 7

1. M Simpson, R Buckman, M Stewart. *Doctor-Patient Communication: the Toronto consensus statement.* British Medical Journal 1991

2. W Stewart. *Counselling in Nursing.* Harper & Row 1983

3. Clemence **Due,** Stephanie Chiarolli,and Damien W. Riggs. *The Impact of pregnancy loss on Men's Health and Wellbeing : A systematic review.* BMC Pregnancy Childbirth. Published online Nov 15th; 17: 380. 2017

4. Terry Maguire: *Why didn't anyone ask if I was OK? Miscarriage Report: Dads grieve too.* Daily Telegraph: 22 July 2014

5. S Gameiro, J Bolvin, L Peronace, C Verhaak. *Why do patients discontinue fertility treatment? A Systematic review of reasons and predictors of discontinuation in fertility treatment.* Human Reproductive Update, November 2012

6. A Huppelschoten *et al. Improving patient-centredness of fertility care using a multifaceted approach.* Biomed Central (BMC) open access 2012

7. E Haagen. *Subfertile couples' negative experiences with uterine insemination care.* Family Practitioner, 2008

8. E Dancet *et al. Patient Centred Infertility Care: a qualitative study to listen to the patient's voice.* Human Reproduction, April 2011

9. *Promoting Cultural Diversity and Cultural Competency: Self-Assessment Checklist For Personnel Providing Services and Supports to Individuals and Families Affected by Sudden and Unexpected Infant Death (SUID)* NCCC Georgetown University On-line

10. Kimberley R Monden *et al. Delivering bad news to Patients.* Baylor University Medical Center Jan 29(1): 101-102 2016

11. Walter F Baile *et al. SPIKES - A Six- step Protocol for Delivering Bad News : Application to The Patient with Cancer.* The Oncologist vol. 5 no. 4 302-311, August 2000

12. Pauline McCulloch. *The patient experience of receiving bad news from health professionals.* Nursing Times January 2004

13. Roberts L R *et al. Social and cultural factors associated with perinatal grief in Chhattisgarh, India.* J Community Health. 2012;37(3):572–582. doi:10.1007/s10900-011-9485-0

14. Jodi Shaefer. *Bulletin for the National Fetal and Infant Mortality Review Program,* July 2007

# CHAPTER 8

1.  Salehi K, Kohan S. Maternal-fetal attachment: what we know and what we need to know. Int J Pregn & Chi Birth. 2017;2(5):146-148. DOI: 10.15406/ipcb.2017.02.00038

2.  Sadat Sadeghi, Mansoureh; Mazaheri, Ali. *Attachment styles in mothers with or without abortions.* Medical Journal of Reproduction & Infertility; Tehran Vol. 8, Iss. 1, 60-69. 2007

3.  Cecily Begley. *I cried ... I had to ... student midwives' experience of stillbirth, miscarriage and neonatal death.* Evidence Based Midwifery. RCM 2009

4.  *Promoting Cultural Diversity and Cultural Competency: Self-Assessment Checklist for Personnel Providing Services and Supports to Individuals and Families Affected by Sudden and Unexpected Infant Death (SUID) NCCC* Georgetown University On-line

Printed in Poland
by Amazon Fulfillment
Poland Sp. z o.o., Wrocław

61468316R00106